Community Health Care in Cuba

Also Available from Lyceum Books, Inc.

Community Health Care in Cuba

EDITED BY

Susan E. Mason
Yeshiva University
Wurzweiler School of Social Work

David L. Strug
Yeshiva University
Wurzweiler School of Social Work

Joan Beder
Yeshiva University
Wurzweiler School of Social Work

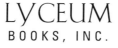

LYCEUM
BOOKS, INC.

Chicago, Illinois

© Lyceum Books, Inc., 2010

Published by

LYCEUM BOOKS, INC.
5758 S. Blackstone Ave.
Chicago, Illinois 60637
773+643-1903 (Fax)
773+643-1902 (Phone)
lyceum@lyceumbooks.com
http://www.lyceumbooks.com

6 5 4 3 2 1   10 11 12 13

ISBN 978-1-933478-72-2

Library of Congress Cataloging-in-Publication Data

Community health care in Cuba / edited by Susan Mason, David Strug, Joan Beder.
   p. cm.
Includes bibliographical references and index.
ISBN 978-1-933478-72-2 (alk. paper)
 1. Community health services—Cuba. I. Mason, Susan Elizabeth. II. Strug, David L.
III. Beder, Joan, 1944–
   RA456.C7C66   2010
   362.1097291—dc22
                                                              2009005099

To the health-care workers of Cuba

CUBA 2009

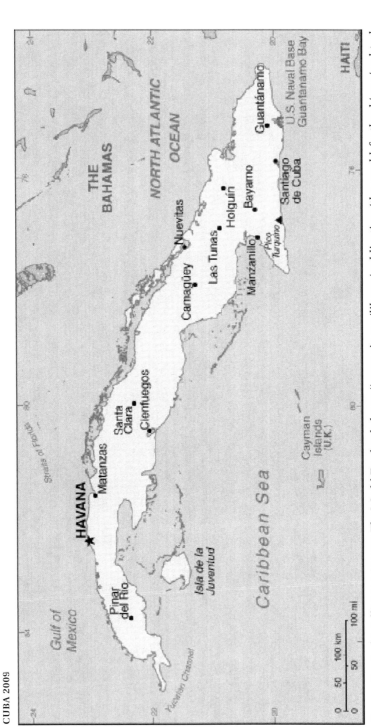

Source: Central Intelligence Agency, The World Factbook, https://www.cia.gov/library/publications/the-world-factbook/geos/cu.html

Contents

Preface

Community Health Care in Cuba describes Cuba's unique, integrated health-care system and examines health care at the local community level using an ecological perspective. It discusses neighborhood consultation centers, municipal polyclinics, tertiary medical facilities, and specialized interventions for people with severe and chronic mental illness, dementia, breast cancer, HIV/AIDS, and other health-care problems. It describes health-care interventions for Cubans of different ages, including children, adolescents, and the elderly.

This edited volume is the result of the research we conducted on health care in Cuba over a number of years as well as the research of other North American and Cuban experts who contributed important chapters. We have had the opportunity as faculty members of the Wurzweiler School of Social Work at Yeshiva University in New York City to travel to Cuba between 2001 and 2007 to conduct research on various aspects of the Cuban health-care system. This included an investigation carried out in December 2005 in Havana with faculty from the Department of Family and Social Medicine at Yeshiva University's Albert Einstein College of Medicine. This research was sponsored by MEDICC (Medical Education Cooperation with Cuba), a nonprofit organization working to enhance cooperation among the U.S., Cuban, and global health communities.

The purpose of *Community Health Care in Cuba* is to familiarize readers with Cuba's highly successful, integrated, and prevention-oriented health-care model through a detailed discussion of health-care delivery from the local to the national levels. Primary medical care is available to all Cubans, resulting in health statistics that are often better than or equal to those of nations that have far more resources. Cuba guarantees to all citizens education and health care, which is delivered with the help of an intricate infrastructure. While the system is not perfect, it encompasses the basic health doctrine in Cuba's culture, that staying healthy is the responsibility of all its citizens. Like that of any other country, Cuba's health system responds to both economic fluctuations and political necessities. Nevertheless, there is an ongoing national commitment for an exemplary health system that begins and, for the most part, remains in the community. The information that is available to investigators outside Cuba suggests that the life expectancy in Cuba will soon near eighty years. That Cuba is able to gain so much health advantage from very limited resources suggests that there are lessons to be learned here for all countries, including the United States, and especially for developing nations with scarce resources.

This volume describes the "intersectorial" nature of the Cuban health-care system, which incorporates nonmedical health determinants including employment, nutrition, sports, culture, education, and housing. As one of our authors (Spiegel, chapter 10) notes about the Cuban health-care system, a "space" exists in health councils at national, provincial, municipal, and local levels for health to be explicitly integrated with other sectors.

The community-oriented nature of the Cuban health-care system is described throughout the book. Family doctor/nurse teams located throughout the community are at the heart of community health care in Cuba. Primary care providers in the neighborhood work closely with polyclinics, which represent a secondary level of care at the municipal level. These primary health-care teams also work closely with hospitals, which represent a tertiary level of care. Many chapters show that these primary, secondary, and tertiary levels are well integrated with one another. They note that Cuba's governmental structure encourages community members to work together with health professionals to improve the well-being of the community. It can be said that Cubans are proud of their health system and that it is a national achievement.

Each chapter in *Community Health Care in Cuba* makes use of principles from social ecology to describe the delivery and use of health care, in particular at the community level. Social ecology refers to the interrelationship between human beings and their social environment. By extension, it applies to the relationship of community to the wider society. Social ecology, however, serves only as a template; the chapters discuss multiple ways of explaining the growth and evolution of the Cuban health system, including other theoretical perspectives.

Community Health Care in Cuba is divided into six parts. The chapters in each section are grounded in data collected and analyzed by their authors, highly respected professionals in the health field and in the social sciences who either live in Cuba or have traveled there.

Part I provides an overview of the Cuban health-care system. This includes a chapter by Susan Mason on the history of Cuban health care prior to the revolution of 1959. She notes that between 1959 and 1963, one-third of Cuban physicians left the country and that those who stayed worked for the new revolutionary government to construct the community-based health system that Cuba has today. In the following chapter, David Strug describes the relevance of social ecology to the Cuban health-care system. He notes that an underlying assumption of the principles of social ecology is that service delivery at the local level should be based on an active partnership between outside experts and members of the community. Strug discusses how this applies to community-oriented health care in Cuba. Next, Julie Feinsilver indicates how and why Cuba could and would develop a national health system, how it has evolved, and the role it plays in Cuba's domestic and international politics.

This part also includes a chapter on medical education that is coauthored by Matthew Anderson of the Albert Einstein College of Medicine in New York City and public-health researcher and medical historian Enrique Beldarraín Chaple of Cuba's National School of Public Health. They note that the Cuban medical system has been remarkably successful in terms of training health-care personnel and that by 2005 there were more than 70,000 physicians working in Cuba; this contrasts with 6,300 in 1959.

Pedro Urra, the founder and director of Cuba's medical information network (INFOMED) explains in an interview with the editors how INFOMED is aligned with Cuban health strategies that place a priority on community medicine through an in-depth and creative use of information and communication technologies. Enrique Beldarraín Chaple's chapter on the history of primary care in Cuba rounds out part I. He notes that Cuba designed and developed its national health system starting in 1959 with the fundamental principles that would allow it to achieve the results advanced in the now famous World Health Organization (WHO) international conference on primary health care held in Alma-Ata in the former Soviet Union. This conference, held in 1978, proposed a strategy for the development of primary care and aimed at achieving universally accessible health care for individuals and families in the community through their full participation. Beldarraín Chaple asserts that Cuba reached this goal in 1983.

Part II is about medical care in today's Cuba. Joan Beder describes the Cuban Ministry of Public Health's efforts to control cancer, and breast cancer in particular. She describes the work done by Cuba's National Cancer Program to stimulate and support community activism on behalf of breast cancer. Next, Robert Fortner discusses the Cuban national program for chronic kidney disease. He explains that the National Program for Chronic Renal Disease Dialysis, and Renal Transplantation is a multitiered effort fully integrated into the national Cuban health system, which is prevention-oriented and aimed at early detection and management of diseases that can lead to kidney failure. Susan Mason explores the history of care for those afflicted with HIV/AIDS, with particular emphasis on efforts toward prevention initiated by the Cuban health-care system. Jerry Spiegel, director of the Centre for International Health at the University of British Columbia, examines how efforts to meet the health needs of Cubans have included systematic processes targeting the determinants of health to promote equity. He notes that this approach reflects the underpinnings of basic policy, including "intersectorality" and "community capacity."

Part III discusses social work and health care in Cuba. This part includes an interview with Odalys González Jubán, president of the Cuban Society for Social Workers in Health Care. Social workers in health care play a major role in assisting people in both urban and rural settings to obtain social services, especially those with health problems. Strug and Odalys González Jubán note that social workers in health care collaborate closely with other health-care professionals and function at all levels of the national health-care system. González Jubán describes her work at a municipal polyclinic and describes its intersecting and interdisciplinary nature. The next chapter is on caring for those with dementia. Wendy Hulko of Thompson Rivers University in Kamloops, British Columbia, and Niurka Cascudo Barral of the Cuban Research Center on Longevity, Aging and Health in Havana, describe care for community-dwelling adults with dementia. They note that Cuba has one of the fastest-aging populations in the developing world and that the health-care system's ongoing attention in the community to elderly persons with and without dementia reduces the cost of prolonged medical care, helps to avoid crises, and ensures that the needs of older adults will be discovered and addressed. David Strug writes about the frail elderly in Cuba and the assistance that social workers provide this population. He notes how social workers access social relationships and the ties and networks among neighbors, community organizations, and health professionals (social capital) to help the frail elderly obtain health care and social assistance.

Part IV focuses on mental health, psychology, and music therapy as a mental-health intervention. Susan Mason's chapter on mental-health care for adolescents notes that it is impossible to describe mental-health treatment in Cuba apart from the societal and ideological forces that permeate the country and bring about basic conflicts. This applies to adolescents in whom the ideals of the revolution are cherished but who also wish for a more open and individualized society. Mason writes that this conflict in values brings special challenges to adolescents in their journey toward adulthood, which mental-health specialists need to consider. In a subsequent chapter on mental-health care and concerns, she describes Cuba's community model of mental-health care, where the community participates in creating programs that support good mental health. Psychologist Jeanne Parr Lemkau's chapter on psychology in Cuba describes what she has learned about the involvement of psychologists in community work in Cuba, based on her multiple trips to the island. She notes that community interventions are structured to achieve two goals: to prevent mental illness and to contain symptoms once they have occurred. The final chapter in this section is about music therapy by music therapist and researcher Melanie Nevis. She notes that music is an integral part of life in Cuba and represents a crucial aspect of Cuban cultural identity and pride. Nevis discusses the cultural and historical use of music as a therapeutic or healing modality in Cuban culture, current developments in music therapy in Cuba, and her research and intercultural collaboration with mental-health communities in Cuba.

Part V describes health-related issues in Cuba's Jewish, Afro-American, and Chinese-Cuban communities. The chapter on the Jewish community written by Strug, Sweifach, and Heft LaPorte focuses on medical assistance and health-promotion programs that are funded and supported by international Jewish organizations. The authors note that these organizations promote family cohesion and have a positive influence on the general well-being of Jewish community members, in addition to providing medical aid. Wong's discussion of the challenges felt by the now-small Chinese community in their efforts to retain their health culture focuses on self-healing. Faguagua Iglesias describes the mindset of Afro-Cuban women, who live in a world in which gender and racial realities conflict with the government's policy of equality for all, including in health care.

In part VI, Grisell Pérez Hoz, an associate professor at the Higher Institute of Medical Sciences in Havana, describes Cuba's achievements in promoting international health, in her chapter on Cuba's medical cooperation with other countries.

The chapters in this volume provide a detailed description of health care in Cuba as it existed up to the time the contributors wrote their chapters. Most recently, modifications to some aspects of the Cuban health-care system are being considered in light of changes in Cuba since the time that former President Fidel Castro left office. However, the community-oriented health care model described in the chapters of this book remains in place.

Acknowledgments

We would like to acknowledge the following people for their generous contributions of time and effort that made this book possible: Sheldon Gelman, PhD, dean of the Wurzweiler School of Social Work, Yeshiva University, and Morton Lowengrub, PhD, provost of Yeshiva University, both of whom believed in our work and provided generous support. We would also like to thank Diane Appelbaum, RN, U.S. director of MEDICC; Michele Frank, MD; Dolly Sacristan, MSW, of Wurzweiler, who helped us with e-mails and translations; Albert S. Kuperman, PhD, associate dean of Medical Education, Albert Einstein School of Medicine, Yeshiva University, who helped us begin our visits that resulted in this book; the Department of Social Medicine of the Albert Einstein College of Medicine; the faculty and staff at the National School of Public Health of Cuba; the Cuban Society of Social Workers in Health Care; the Social Work Faculty at the University of Havana; the members of the Breast Cancer Program for Cuban Women (Wings for Life); the psychologists and psychiatrists who provided invaluable information; and our Cuban translators.

We would also like to thank our family members, without whose support we could not have completed this project.

Contributor Biographies

Matthew Anderson
Matthew Anderson is a native of New York City. He is a family physician working at Montefiore Medical Center in the Bronx and assistant professor of family and social medicine at Albert Einstein College of Medicine. He has lived and worked overseas, mostly notably in Haiti and Guatemala. He has a long relationship with one of the main AIDS clinics in Guatemala City, where he worked as a Fulbright Scholar in 1999. He is coeditor of the bilingual online journal Social Medicine (www.socialmedicine.info), published in association with the Latin American Social Medicine Association (ALAMES). He is also coeditor of the Social Medicine Portal (www.socialmedicine.org) a Web site devoted to promoting social medicine.

Niurka Cascudo Barral
Niurka Cascudo Barral, MD, graduated with honors in medicine from the Salvador Allende Medical Faculty. She is a specialist in both family and geriatric medicine. Niurka Cascudo Barral has postgraduate training in Satisfactory Longevity, which is a gerontological training program in Cuba aimed at improving the lives of older persons. She is chief of Diagnostic Consultation for Cognitive Deterioration at the Ibero-American Center for the Third Age in Havana.

Joan Beder
Joan Beder is professor of social work at the Wurzweiler School of Social Work at Yeshiva University in New York City and maintains a clinical practice in Long Island. Much of her research and writing has been focused on medical issues, death and dying, and bereavement. Recent research has focused on social workers who work in the military. She has presented at numerous conferences, both national and international,

on a variety of topics related to her research interests. She is the author of *Faces of Bereavement: A Casebook for Grief Counselors* and *Medical Social Work: The Interface of Medicine and Caring.* She has traveled several times to Cuba as part of a group to do research on health care with particular interest in the care of the breast cancer population.

Enrique Beldarraín Chaple

Enrique Beldarraín Chaple, MD, received his doctorate in medicine in 1982 at the Superior Institute of Medical Sciences in Havana. He holds a degree in epidemiology from the Faculty of Public Health of the National School of Public Health. He has conducted research in medical anthropology, is professor of information management, and auxiliary professor in the history of medicine at the National School of Public Health. He has published four books. His latest book, *Doctors and the Beginning of Anthropology in Cuba*, won a prestigious prize from the Cuban Academy of Sciences in 2007. He has published more than thirty articles in Cuban and foreign professional journals and has been invited to lecture at universities in Latin America, Europe, and the United States.

Julie Feinsilver

Julie Feinsilver has published extensively on Cuba, including the book, *Healing the Masses: Cuban Health Politics At Home and Abroad* and articles and book chapters on Cuban domestic policies and foreign affairs, biotechnology, and nontraditional exports. Her work on Cuban medical diplomacy has been published in *Foreign Affairs en Español* (Oct.–Dec. 2006) and *Nueva Sociedad* (July–Aug. 2008). Two book chapters on different aspects of Cuban medical diplomacy are forthcoming in 2009. She is currently visiting researcher at the Center for Latin American Studies at Georgetown University.

Robert W. Fortner

Robert W. Fortner, MD, graduated from the University of Washington School of Medicine in 1967, interned at Los Angeles County Hospital, and completed residency and fellowship training at Walter Reed Army Medical Center. He served as chief of the Nephrology Service at William Beaumont Army Medical Center from 1971 to 1973. As director of the hemodialysis program at El Camino Hospital in Mountain View, California, he championed home hemodialysis as the treatment modality of choice for end-stage renal disease, and El Camino Dialysis Services became the largest home-dialysis provider in the state. Dr. Fortner assembled a team, funded by grants from Medicare, that collaborated on the development of a "Capitated Payment System for all ESRD services," a version of which is now being tested by others. Relocating to Bainbridge Island, Washington, in 1989, he has continued to work as a consultant, while pursuing other interests. He traveled to Cuba in 2006 for Atlantic Philanthropies to examine the Cuban nephrology program.

Grisell Pérez Hoz

Grisell Pérez Hoz holds a bachelor's degree in education from the Pablo Lafargue Superior Institute of Pedagogy and a master's degree (MSc) in Higher Medical Education from the National School of Public Health in Cuba. She is associate professor at the Higher Institute of Medical Sciences and at the National School of Public Health in Havana. She has participated as a course leader in more than thirty international public-health courses for undergraduate and postgraduate foreign students from different countries, including Ecuador, Mexico, Sweden, Great Britain, and the United States.

Wendy Hulko

Wendy Hulko is assistant professor of social work at Thompson Rivers University in Kamloops, British Columbia, and a qualified health researcher with the Centre for Research on Personhood in Dementia (CRPD) at the University of British Columbia in Vancouver. She holds a BA Hon. in sociology and Spanish (Trent University), an MSW (University of Toronto), and a PhD in sociology and social policy (University of Stirling) and has worked in the field of gerontology since 1993. Her experience includes long-term care nursing, hospital social work, life history and dementia research, government policy and planning (health and aging), and community development. She met her coauthor Dr. Niurka Cascudo Barral while a student doing research in Cuba, and their collaboration led her to bring a group of Canadian social work students to the Ibero-American Center for the Third Age in 2008, as part of a field school on Cuban approaches to health and social welfare.

María Ileana Faguagua Iglesias

María Ileana Faguagua Iglesias is a Cuban anthropologist. She holds a *licentiate* degree in history from the University of Havana, a master's degree in anthropology from the University of Havana and the Fundación Fernando Ortíz, and a diplomate in ethnology from the Fundación Fernando Ortíz. She is the Cuban director of the Inter-Cultural and Inter-religious Program for Dialog of the Commission for the Study of the History of the Church in Latin America. She has conducted research on the interracial relations in Cuba and on Afro-Cuban women, among other topics.

Odalys González Jubán

Odalys González Jubán is president of the Cuban Society of Social Workers in Health Care. She holds the degree of *Licenciatura* in the technology of health with a specialty in social and occupational rehabilitation.

Heidi Heft LaPorte

Heidi Heft LaPorte is associate professor in social work at Lehman College, City University of New York. She teaches qualitative and quantitative research methods, single-system design/practice evaluation research, social welfare organization, and human behavior in the social environment. In addition to her research on Jewish identity and identification among Cuban Jews living both inside and outside of Cuba, Heft LaPorte has carried out research in a variety of areas, including HIV/AIDS, domestic violence, child welfare, workforce training, group work, computer technology and social work practice in hospital and case management settings, social work educational objectives, and outcomes and curriculum innovations.

Jeanne Parr Lemkau

Jeanne Parr Lemkau is a psychologist, writer, and professor emerita of family medicine and community health at Wright State University School of Medicine in Dayton, Ohio. She holds a doctorate in clinical psychology and a master's degree in creative nonfiction writing. In the early 1970s, she served with the Peace Corps in rural Nicaragua. Subsequently, as a faculty member in family medicine, she developed curricula in global health, led medical delegations to Nicaragua, and studied and taught about health care in Cuba. Since 2000, she has traveled to Cuba on research, educational, and humanitarian trips seven times. She has published widely on cultural issues, psychology, and family medicine, and recently collaborated with David Strug of Yeshiva University on a study of the effects of travel restrictions on Cuban-American families. In 2006, she organized and, with Strug, wrote *Love, Loss, and Longing: The Impact of U.S. Travel Policy on Cuban-American Families,* a photography exhibit that toured nationally and was published as a book by the Latin America Working Group and the Washington Office on Latin America. She practices clinical psychology and writes in Yellow Springs, Ohio.

Susan E. Mason

Susan E. Mason is professor of social work at Yeshiva University's Wurzweiler School of Social Work and professor of sociology and chair of the college departments of sociology and political science. She holds a doctorate in sociology and education and a social work degree from Columbia University as well as graduate degrees from New York University and the University of Chicago. Mason has authored more than forty peer-reviewed articles and book chapters that mostly focus on mental health, social service utilization, and workforce efficacy. She is coeditor of *Diagnosis Schizophrenia, A Comprehensive Resource for Patients, Families and Helping Professionals.* She has traveled to Cuba numerous times to conduct research for this book.

Melanie Nevis

Melanie Nevis has a master's degree in music therapy from New York University. She is the director of music therapy at the Brooklyn/Queens Conservatory of Music in Brooklyn, and is the founder and director of Healing Connections, an international music therapy organization providing music therapy services, training, research, and consultation. Nevis has also completed training in Gestalt therapy at the Gestalt International Study Center in Wellfleet, Massachusetts. A specialist in percussion-based music therapy, she received a grant from the Tinker Foundation for research on "The Therapeutic Aspects of Cuban Folkloric Drumming," which contributed to her thesis on "Influences of Afro-Cuban Drumming Traditions on Percussion-Based Music Therapy." She has studied, taught, and conducted research in Cuba since 1994.

Jerry Spiegel

Jerry Spiegel (MA, MSc, PhD) is director of global health at the Liu Institute for Global Issues, associate professor of health care and epidemiology and director of the Centre for International Health at the University of British Columbia, and has been involved in collaborative research and teaching programs in Cuba since the mid-1990s. He is a Michael Smith Foundation for Health Research scholar and Canadian Institutes for Health Research Institute for Population and Public Health new investigator. He is also past (and founding) president of the Canadian Coalition for Global Health Research and cochair of its Research to Action Task Group. He currently directs research programs on globalization, social organization and health, and the ecosystem approach to human health and vulnerable populations. In addition to his work in Cuba, where he has published extensively with Cuban colleagues, he is also conducting research and training programs in Mexico and Ecuador on effective "intersectoral" and transdisciplinary methods for managing environmental health risks. Specific investigations have explored matters such as the impacts of tourism development on gender and health in coastal communities, sustainable prevention and control of dengue, and ways to strengthen the capacity of universities to work effectively with communities and other stakeholders.

David L. Strug

David L. Strug is professor of social work at the Wurzweiler School of Social Work at Yeshiva University in New York City and is also a clinical social worker in private practice. He received his PhD in anthropology from Columbia University, his MSW from the Hunter College School of Social Work, and his MPH from the University of California at Berkeley. He has traveled to Cuba frequently in recent years, where he has conducted research on older persons, on the development of social work, and on community-oriented health care. David Strug is the coauthor with Jeanne Lemkau of *Love, Loss and Longing: The Impact of U.S. Travel Restrictions on Cuban-American Families.*

Jay Sweifach

Jay Sweifach is associate professor at the Wurzweiler School of Social Work at Yeshiva University in New York City. He has an extensive list of authored and coauthored papers that have been published in leading social work and interdisciplinary journals. He has presented at academic conferences both nationally and internationally on topics including domestic violence, social work education, ethics, sex education, and volunteerism.

Pedro Urra

Pedro Urra is the director of the National Medical Sciences Information Center and the founder and director of INFOMED. Urra is a full adjunct professor of information technologies at the University of Havana's School of Library and Information Sciences. He has dedicated his professional career to information management, the development of the national virtual health infrastructure, and the training of human resources in health information. He helped to develop the Latin American and Caribbean Virtual Health Library and the Virtual Health University.

Joyce Wong

Joyce Wong graduated from the Columbia University School of Social Work and has been working as a social worker with the Southeast Asian community in the Bronx, New York, for nearly two decades, providing out-patient mental-health services at Montefiore Hospital Department of Psychiatry/Family Medicine. She has taught as an adjunct professor at the Hunter College School of Social Work and has been involved in training medical students and family-practice residents on refugee mental health. Most recently, she traveled to Italy to participate in a certificate program on Global Mental Health: Trauma and Recovery by the Harvard Program in Refugee Trauma.

PART I

Introduction and Overview of the Cuban Health-Care System

CHAPTER ONE

Cuban Health Care Prior to the 1959 Revolution

Susan E. Mason

Cuban history is rich with stories of internal struggles and challenges from both successful and would-be conquerors. From colonial Cuba, through the wars of independence, the early republic, and until the fall of Fulgencio Batista's dictatorship that ended with the 1959 revolution, health and health concerns were an important theme that became central in Fidel Castro's Cuba. A brief review of health concerns before 1959 provides a useful backdrop for understanding the current health system.

Disease and the Response to it in Early Cuba

Columbus came to Cuba in 1492 and declared it a part of the Spanish Empire. Over the next century, a variety of Spanish conquistadores made stops in Cuba to solidify Spain's hold on the island, but most did not stay long. When only small amounts of gold were found, Cuba became a way station for the more lucrative expeditions to North and South America. Havana developed as the main city toward the end of the sixteenth century, when its harbor was used as the fueling station for ships bound for Spain, other parts of the Caribbean, and the Americas. During most of the sixteenth century, the Spanish and first generation Cubans, called Creoles, vanquished the indigenous population, the

Tainos, Ciboneys, and Guanajatabeyes. These native peoples, once making up a population of about 112,000, were forced to work for the Spanish under the harshest of conditions. They worked in the mines, on the farms, and in menial jobs in the villages and cities. It is estimated that by the mid-1500s their numbers were reduced from 112,000 in pre-Columbian times to about 3,000 through starvation, overwork, disease, and suicide (Perez, 2006).

The Spanish brought starvation to the native people, whose food supply had been primarily derived from the land. Throughout the 1500s, native Cuban farmlands were overrun with wild pigs and other animals brought in by the Spanish, to such an extent that whole communities starved with little recourse (Perez, 2006). Disease took a huge toll as well. Diseases brought from Europe such as smallpox, typhus, influenza, and measles frequently led to death for people without immunity to them. Influenza and the common cold were especially deadly, often causing bronchial pneumonia, for which the native population had no resistance (Staten, 2003). Overwork of indigenous people forced to work on farms, ships, in mines, and everywhere there was a need for hard labor contributed to the decimation of the population. Native people were literally distributed to the Spanish under the *encomienda* system, where workers in effect belonged to the land, much as in feudal Europe. Long hours of work coupled with routine abuse led to early deaths and few births (Perez, 2006).

Suicide among the native Cubans was perhaps the most disturbing result of Spanish maltreatment, with an estimated 35 percent of all indigenous people choosing to take their own lives. Stories of natives desperate to die by eating dirt and taking poisons were common in the sixteenth century. In one village, as many as fifty inhabitants were found hanged, including women and children. The Spanish response was to either torture or kill those who had not succeeded in killing themselves. This did little to stem the tide, and in later chronicles of Cuban history, suicide was known as the way vulnerable groups protested oppressors. It became a form of protest carried out by African slaves, Chinese laborers, and Cuban revolutionaries fighting Spain and later the Batista regime prior to the 1959 revolution (Perez, 2005).

Colonial Health and African Slavery

With few exceptions, the early Spanish settlers came to Cuba without women. As European women were scarce on the island, indigenous women were taken as concubines, producing generations of Creoles with part-native blood. Creoles also had children with African slaves, whose offspring were customarily declared free, creating a large wage-earning mulatto population that worked mainly in the cities. The Creoles focused on getting rich through exploiting the land and using available cheap labor. When it became clear that there were not enough indigenous people to exploit, Africans, as slaves, were forced to work in the gold and copper mines and on the farms. African slave importation began slowly but increased in the mid-1700s through trade with the English slave agents. By 1860 there were an estimated three hundred thousand to four hundred thousand African slaves in Cuba, who mostly worked on the sugar and tobacco farms but also in the cities, providing services to the Creoles. Working conditions for African slaves were horribly harsh, and they too succumbed to disease and exhaustion. The forced-labor Africans lived in barracks in crowded, unsanitary conditions that brought about large numbers of deaths from infectious diseases. The mortality rate was estimated to be 10 to 12 percent a year (Perez, 2006). Slave importation continued into the 1860s, long after Spain declared the trade to be illegal in 1820. With the end of slavery in the United States in 1865 and the failed ten-year war that the Creoles conducted beginning in 1868 for liberation from Spain, the illegal slave trade—but not slavery—was brought to a conclusion. Slaves were freed gradually in Cuba from the 1870s to the 1880s, but they were often forced to continue their work on farms for very low wages and to live in conditions conducive to disease and early death (Perez, 2006).

Early Rural Health Care

Medical attention in the early years in rural Cuba was often left to native healers for the indigenous people and African healers for the slaves. For the Creoles there were the barbers, who acted as bleeders and dentists. Bleeding was the accepted form of reducing fevers until the mid to late nineteenth century. Midwives and bonesetters were available for all population groups. Very few licensed physicians practiced in Cuba, and this was especially true in the rural areas; small infirmaries, *casas de salud*, were common in the villages but had few licensed doctors. Wealthy Creoles who became ill often went to the cities to obtain care, to Havana in the west and to Santiago in the east. The curative success rates for the physicians in the years before the late nineteenth century were not higher than those of the local practitioners (Danielson, 1979).

Health Concerns in the Early Cities and Surrounding Countryside

Cities developed beginning in the late 1500s and attracted a diverse group of workers providing services to the Creole population, who looked to the cities as centers of trade and culture. Havana was established in the northwest and Santiago in the southeast. Free Africans from other islands came to Cuba's cities to work and were joined by the remaining indigenous groups and new immigrants from Europe and from other Caribbean islands. The Creoles were in competition with the *peninsulares,* or immigrants from Spain, who were granted government jobs, land, and special privileges, Spain's way of retaining loyalty on the island. The government in Spain thought that by sending people to Cuba they would stabilize the population and retain their hold on the colony. This created two classes of "white" people who often competed for the same resources and who, with diverse interests, rarely considered the well-being of other population groups. Single immigrant men from Spain and elsewhere in Europe, who did not work the farms, settled in the cities along with others from Spain who were using cities, mostly Havana, as a way station before traveling to other destinations. Havana, as the major port, added these *peninsulares* and other European whites to its already crowded housing conditions, and although this group lived in the better areas, their simple presence was an important factor in the spread of disease (Gott, 2004). Freed slaves, indigenous people, recent poor immigrants, and a substantial number of Spanish ex-soldiers without means lived in the slums and shantytowns in and around Havana and other cities. On the outskirts of the cities and in the poor villages near farms, day laborers lived in less than ideal conditions that became breeding grounds for disease. The few available physicians in the countryside and folk healers had few remedies for most infectious diseases.

Not all city dwellers were poor. There are records of free Africans with skills who earned relatively high wages and lived in the better neighborhoods. Many were trained as physician's helpers and even as physicians, although they were unable to obtain licenses and were barred from the better medical facilities (Danielson, 1979; Perez, 2006). Still, the poor sanitation of the slum areas affected all city residents, and diseases such as yellow fever, tuberculosis, smallpox, and measles were reported to take large tolls. Wealthy Creoles left the cities to the relative safety of the countryside when epidemics broke out. The poor city workers stayed and tried to survive on meager nutrition and in unsanitary conditions. In the countryside, the ex-slaves and other laborers did not fare much better.

As late as the mid-nineteenth century, African slaves and the Chinese immigrants who slowly replaced them as cheap labor suffered early deaths from work exhaustion. Family life was initially discouraged for the Africans, the indigenous groups, and the Chinese. The Creole practice of importing mostly African male slaves, thinking that it was too expensive to support families and raise children, created an imbalance in the population. Indigenous women were in short supply to the indigenous men because of their roles as concubines for the Creoles. Chinese workers were mostly men. It is suggested that this general lack of family life contributed to the high suicide rates and psychological and emotional states of depression that have been pervasive throughout Cuban history (Perez, 2005).

Medical Training

Medical training in the colonies was limited to clinical training at hospitals and courses at the University of Havana. The university was founded for religious training in 1768 and provided limited training to Creole students until 1834, when it added its medical department. Medical licenses were granted through the *Protomedicato*, the licensing board that required applicants to have medical training that included supervised work with patients, faith in Catholicism, and a good character. Licensed physicians competed with unlicensed doctors, healers, and barbers, who were widely acknowledged to be the island's dentists. Licensed doctors, or *protophysicans* as they were called, were assigned territories by the *Protomedicato* and were obligated to serve the poor, but largely doctored only those who could pay. Their numbers were few; by the end of the eighteenth century, there were only a hundred in all of Cuba, and they served mostly the white population. Mulattos, free Africans, slaves, and indigenous people were served by folk doctors, phlebotomists, herbalists, and pseudo-pharmacists known as *boticarios*, or *droguistas* (Danielson, 1979).

Records of disease outbreaks were formalized in most cities in the early 1800s, and in 1804 the Vaccination Board was established in Havana to prevent the spread of smallpox. The pioneering physician Dr. Tomás Romay y Chacón was largely responsible for the introduction and distribution of the smallpox vaccine in Cuba. He also promoted and later influenced the secularization of medical education, wherein medical students would not have to be Catholic to be admitted to schools and later licensed. Later in the century, Dr. Carlos Finlay, who could not gain admission to the University of Havana because of his modest social background, studied medicine in the United States and returned to Cuba to prove that yellow fever was caused by mosquitoes. This discovery led to yellow fever inoculations that virtually eliminated the disease by 1901. Public water filtration was introduced in Havana in the 1870s to help fight dysentery and cholera caused by poor sanitation (Danielson, 1979).

Most of the health advances took place in the cities, most notably in Havana. The western section of Cuba, where Havana is located, became its commercial and cultural center. The eastern section was largely made up of small farms and sugar mills, and Santiago, its largest city, fell behind Havana in population and development.

The Role of Hospitals

Hospitals were first established for the military in the late 1500s and by 1600 there were small hospitals in Havana, Santiago, and Bayamo (Danielson, 1979). People in other cities were mostly served by the military hospitals that offered care to the general population in separate wards. Gradually, a small number of specialty hospitals were added; there were several for women, two leprosy hospitals, and an insane asylum that began in Havana in 1834. Hospitals throughout the cities and in the countryside were staffed by royal or state-owned slaves, free Africans, older mulatto women, and wealthy Creole women who attended to the poor as an act of charity. In the small dispensaries in the countryside, medical care for Creoles was dispensed by physicians and surgeons who were often unlicensed, many of whom had informal medical education.

Hospitals were mostly avoided by wealthy Creoles, who preferred to seek medical attention in their own homes or homes rented for sick care. Hospitals such as San Ambrosio in Havana in the late 1700s had separate wards to treat military personnel, poor immigrants, forced labor including convicts and slaves, free Africans, and poor women about to give birth (Danielson, 1979). Hospital care in Cuba during the eighteenth and up until the mid-nineteenth century was, like elsewhere in the world, no guarantee for recovery. In fact, the opposite was true. Infection rates from surgery and exposure to diseases in hospitals harmed more patients than were helped. The early hospitals did serve as training facilities for physicians and cared for those who could not afford private health services.

The Wars for Independence and Health Care

One of the striking ironies of modern warfare is its tendency to bring about medical advances that later save lives. The wars that Cuba fought for its independence from Spain serve as an example of this phenomenon. The first war for independence began in 1868 and lasted ten years until an uneasy peace was signed in 1878. The second war was fought from 1895 to 1898, when the United States intervened and invaded Cuba. The United States occupied Cuba for four years, when in 1902, failing to get the Cuban population to agree to annexation, its troops were withdrawn, except for the U.S. naval base at Guantánamo, and Cuba became an independent nation for the first time in its history. Politically and economically, Cuba was influenced by the United States, so much so that a substantial number of Cubans wanted the island to be annexed. Those opposing annexation eventually won out, and Cuba later repudiated the 1901 Platt Amendment to the Cuban Constitution that gave the United States the power to intervene for the protection of life and property (Aguilar, 1993).

During the wars there was an increased need for military hospitals, and a large hospital was established in Havana in 1896 that later was used for the civilian population as well. The wars left thousands of people homeless and without family support, resulting in an additional need for health clinics. Small neighborhood clinics developed in the major cities serving this new group of urban adults and children. The wars brought economic ruin to many sugar mill owners and farmers, but physicians found stability by setting up offices in the cities. Mutual aid societies, *quintas*, that offered pre-paid medical plans to immigrants and poor people in general sprung up along with small neighborhood clinics, the *casas de salud*. Although there had been several of these arrangements in earlier years, it was in the late 1800s that these mutualist societies began to take hold in greater numbers (Danielson, 1979).

Yellow fever along with other diseases such as smallpox took thousands of lives during the wars of independence. It is estimated that unsanitary conditions brought on by the Spanish policies that removed farmers from their land to live in disease-ridden sectors of the countryside and in the crowded neighborhoods of the cities caused about 10 percent of the civilian population to perish. Although Carlos J. Finlay announced his discovery of the link between the mosquito and yellow fever in 1881, it was not well-received at first and took twenty years for insect-removal practices to take place. Under the United States occupation, thousands of houses in Havana were made mosquito free, which almost entirely eliminated yellow fever (Danielson, 1979). In Cuba today, schoolchildren spend weekends examining houses for potential mosquito-breeding standing water, an important contribution to the continuation of disease control.

The Triumph of Mutualism

The wars of independence did not bring about lasting peace. Hundreds of thousands of Cubans lost their homes, their wealth, and their places in Cuban society. At the same time, turmoil in Spain led almost three hundred thousand immigrants to arrive in Cuba between the early 1920s and the beginning of World War II. Scarce resources, government corruption, and daily incidents of politically motivated violence were typical in the years after the wars of independence. Internal struggles between various politically leftist and rightist groups and an economy that seemed to be forever in a state of flux contributed to instability. The United States intervened four times with troops between 1898 and 1923 and countless other times with political and economic influence until World War II. After the war, American influence became even greater owing to increasing investments in the Cuban sugar industry. Cuba became the leading exporter of sugar in the world, and as many as half the sugar mills were owned by investors in the United States. Guantánamo, leased from Cuba for $2,000 a year in 1912, remained in U.S. control and still serves as a reminder to Cubans of American influence and interventions in their country (Staten, 2003).

During the period before and directly after World War II, mutualist prepaid health-care organizations served as many as 40 percent of the Cuban population. There were four ways that most Cubans received health services. Large mutual aid groups served the immigrants from Spain and others who identified with Spain as their homeland. Smaller mutual associations served Cubans who could pay modest fees, and fee-for-service private physicians served the wealthy. There were also charity clinics and hospitals that served the poor. Many of these services overlapped at times. Private doctors sometimes used the facilities of the mutualist clinics and the large state/charity hospitals and mutualist subscribers at times used the services of the private physicians. What was clear is that Afro-Cubans were denied access to services that were unofficially designated for whites only. It was not until 1938 that the Transport Workers Union established a mutualist organization, the Centro Benéfico y Juríidico de los Trabajadores de la Habana, which after five years opened its membership to other workers and most importantly had always welcomed nonwhites as members (Danielson, 1979). The popularity of prepaid medical contracts that extended right up until the 1959 revolution was indicative of a culture that accepted the concept of socialized medicine. One important difference was that before the 1959 revolution, the system was fragmented and decentralized. Another difference was the postrevolution focus on extending more services to the rural areas of Cuba, a process that was largely stalled before Fidel Castro took power. An important similarity between the pre- and post-1959 systems is that most medical care took place in the community, although in prerevolutionary Cuba, doctors may not have lived where they worked. In today's Cuba, medical care in the community and in tertiary facilities is free for all people, regardless of ethnicity or race, and physicians are paid salaries by the government. Private medical practice is outlawed.

Urban Versus Rural Medical Services

Cuba's largest city, Havana, undoubtedly had more medical facilities before the 1959 revolution than all the rest of Cuba. Although this still remains true, the present Cuban government has made great strides in equalizing the quantity and quality of services in the rural areas. Physicians are sent to the outlying sectors as part of their community service. Computers link facilities in the provinces with the technical support they may need. All of medical Cuba is linked to INFOMED, a Web site that provides the latest research and linkages to journals, and access to consultations from specialists.

Pre-1959 cities in the eastern sector (Santiago, Bayamo, Camaguey) had fewer medical personnel and resources than western and central Cuba. In the land of the small farmer and small sugar mill, doctors found it difficult to make enough money to live on. Consequently, the less-experienced and even less-qualified doctors practiced in these areas. The statistics of 1934 indicate that the city of Havana had 1,200 physicians, which was almost half the total of the rest of the country's 2,542 physicians. Similarly, Havana's 3,014 hospital beds comprised more than half of the 5,103 found in the rest of the country (Danielson, 1979). The late 1940s and 1950s brought little change in the limited health resources available in rural Cuba. Mutualist plans continued to thrive in the pre-1959 years in the cities. It is estimated that by 1958, half of Havana belonged to a mutualist plan, and in other cities the estimated number of members was 350,000 (Danielson, 1979). Still, these plans were not widespread outside of the cities. Cuban health historian Ross Danielson suggested that urban mutualist plans absorbed so many doctors that they contributed to the lack of doctors serving in rural areas (1979). The doctor-to-population ratio in Havana in the mid-1950s was 1 to 227; but in Oriente, an eastern, largely rural province, it was 1 to 2,423. The post-World War II government under Batista (1952–1959) added to this disparity by directing health funds to Havana and away from other cities and rural areas. The Ministry of Public Health per capita aid to Havana Province was $2.69, but only $0.88 to Oriente (Perez, 2006).

The Revolution in Health Care

At the eve of the socialist revolution, large numbers of Cubans lived in city slums or in shantytowns surrounding the cities. These people were often destitute, and health services were either unavailable or provided on an emergency basis in charity clinics and hospitals. Large numbers of women beggars roamed the streets of Havana with their babies in their arms seeking food from local churches (Perez, 2006), and the possibility of their receiving proper nutrition and medical care was nil. People in the countryside often did not fare better. Most either worked on small farms or for the big sugar estates that were largely financed by investors from the United States. The great majority of rural Cubans relied on whatever health services they could get, and most of it was charity (Staten, 2003). Racial discrimination in both the cities and the countryside still prevailed. Limited health services were available to Afro-Cubans (27 percent of the population by the early 1950s) outside of the few mutualist organizations in the large cities (Danielson, 1979; Perez, 2006).

Between 1959 and 1963, one-third of Cuban physicians left the country, encouraged by the United States to emigrate (Danielson, 1979). Those who stayed worked for the new revolutionary government to construct the community-based health system that Cuba has today.

References

Aguilar, L. (1993). Cuba, c. 1860–c. 1930. In L. Bethell (Ed.), *Cuba: A short history* (pp. 21–56). London: Cambridge University Press.

Danielson, R. (1979). *Cuban medicine*. New Brunswick, NJ: Transaction Books.

Gott, R. (2004). *Cuba, a new history*. New Haven, CT: Yale University Press.

Perez, Jr., L. A. (2005). *To die in Cuba: Suicide and society*. Chapel Hill, NC: University of North Carolina Press.

Perez, Jr., L. A. (2006). *Cuba between reform and revolution, 3rd ed*. New York: Oxford University Press.

Staten, C. L. (2003). *The history of Cuba*. New York: Macmillan.

CHAPTER TWO

Social Ecology and Cuba's Community-Oriented Health-Care System

David L. Strug

Social ecology provides a theoretical perspective for describing Cuba's community-oriented health care system. Social ecology refers to the interrelationship between human beings and their social environment (Bookchin, 1982). By extension, social ecology applies to the relationship of community to the wider society. Beginning with a commitment to optimum health for all citizens, the Cuban health system is grounded in community health care as the foundation for its extensive primary, secondary, and tertiary systems.

The social work academician Michael Ungar (2002) has adapted a number of principles based on the social ecological perspective of Arne Naess (1989), which Ungar extends to practice settings and to the delivery of social services in the community. These principles are easily applied to the health arena. An underlying assumption of these principles is that delivery of services at the local level should be based on an active partnership between outside experts and members of the community. A social ecological perspective in health is in keeping with the Cuban Model of Community-Oriented Primary Care (COPC) approach (Longlett, Kruse, & Wesley, 2001). COPC is a systematic approach to health care based on principles derived from epidemiology, primary care, preventive medicine, and health promotion that has been shown to have positive health benefits for communities (Longlett et al., 2001).

The social ecological practice principles as applied to health are relevant to an understanding of community-oriented health care in Cuba, where health experts at the national, provincial, and municipal levels work together to implement health education, prevention, and treatment in the community. The community, or neighborhood (the two words are used interchangeably), in Cuba is a geographical area that is several square blocks in size and represents an important economic, political, and social unit within society. A municipality is comprised of a number of different communities and is a geographical area from within which a regional level of government operates (Roman, 2003).

Three Principles of Social Ecology

The three features of the social ecology model most relevant to Cuba's approach to health care appear below. They are adapted from Ungar (2002).

PRINCIPLE 1: ALLIANCES OR CONNECTIONS BETWEEN COMMUNITIES AND SERVICES

Structured alliances between communities and services that provide for them act to increase the delivery of resources that are directly available to individuals and families to help them help themselves.

It is important for communities and outside service providers to establish alliances that maximize service delivery to community members and assist them in their ability to help themselves. This principle stands in contrast to the approach in which outside professionals in a hierarchical and bureaucratized system manipulate the community to achieve the goals of the professionals. It represents an alternative vision for structuring alliances between communities and services that allows professionals and community stakeholders to come together at local community institutions such as health clinics and schools, as well as in other important community settings, for the purpose of establishing intervention goals.

An examination of the Cuban health-care system helps us to understand how it facilitates this approach. Health care in Cuba is free and universally accessible at all levels of society, is a basic right of the population, and is prevention oriented. It is decentralized and vertically integrated at the national, provincial, municipal, and community levels (Dresang, Brebrick, Murray, Shallue, & Sullivan-Vedder, 2005). Vertically integrated so that a community-based approach fits with secondary and tertiary levels of care (Pérez-Ávila, 2001), the Cuban health-care system is designed to promote an optimal and rational use of available resources. Each level of care is linked to an appropriate level of government to assist delivery of service and provide accountability.

Cuba's Ministry of Public Health coordinates all levels of health care at the national level. The Cuban health care system has three tiers. Hospital-based care represents one tier, and it exists primarily at the provincial level, with hospitals across the island providing acute-care services.

Polyclinics, dental clinics, homes for at-risk women, centers for the care of the elderly, and other health-care services are organized at the municipal level and represent the second tier of service. A polyclinic is a municipal health-care center that offers many health and social services for nearby community members (Waller, 2002). Cuba's network of more than 470 health-care polyclinics are dedicated to integrating multimedical specialties (e.g., pediatric medicine, heart treatment, ophthalmology, optometry, x-ray, rehabilitation, twenty-four-hour dentistry, minor surgery, ultrasound diagnostics, etc.). In recent years, polyclinics have been modernized in order to increase availability of services to community members and provide many of the services previously available only at hospitals.

Family-medicine consultation centers are located at the community level and represent the third tier of Cuba's three-tiered health-care system. Primary care provided by a family doctor represents a major element of the health-care system at the neighborhood level. Primary care family doctors are the foundation of the Cuban health-care system, and practically all graduates of medical school in Cuba are currently required to complete a family-practice residency. Family doctor/nurse teams provide personalized primary health care to between 125 and 165 families at the block level within the community.

A family-practice office staffed by a doctor/nurse team (*consultorio*) addresses the majority of the health problems in the community and emphasizes health promotion. These teams perform regular home visits and even visit those in good health, thereby offering personalized attention to the individuals and families at greatest risk and facilitating preventive measures (Oficina Nacional de Estadísticas, 1998/1999). The teams consider not only physical health but also examine issues of lifestyle, work life, environment, and nutrition.

The family doctor refers community members to the polyclinic for more specialized care that the doctor cannot directly provide. Family doctors spend a half-day per week joining their patients for specialist visits at the polyclinic. Each family doctor consults with a Basic Working Group (GBT) comprised of internists, podiatrists, and other health-care specialists concerning problematic consultation-center cases. This promotes continuity for patients, builds collegial relationships between family physicians and specialists, and offers education for all parties involved.

Family physicians are required to look at patients in the context of both family and community. The family doctor typically lives in the community in which he or she practices and is viewed as one of its members rather than as an outside health professional coming to work in a poor neighborhood. Community and public health concerns are addressed through neighborhood interventions spearheaded by the family doctor in coordination with community stakeholders. These interventions are coordinated at the municipal level. Community members and their leaders assist the family doctor and nurse in the preparation of an assessment of the health status of the community, which includes a prioritization of neighborhood health issues and a plan of action for the following year.

The Cuban health-care system also incorporates nonmedical health determinants including, employment, nutrition, sports, culture, education, and housing. The government promotes health initiatives through coordination with local decision-making bodies ("people's councils," described below) and through community participation tied to the Healthy Cities movement, promoting greater public involvement in determining health priorities and actions. Through its Healthy Cities program, the Cuban government facilitates the integration of efforts coming from all social and economic sectors of society, thus favoring joint action among these sectors and community members (Spiegel, 2004).

The people's councils (*consejos populares*) represent an important link in Cuba's three-tiered health-care system. They function at a level that is between the municipality and the neighborhood and bridge decision making between the local community and the wider municipal level. A people's council is comprised of community delegates and representatives of grassroots organizations, state enterprises, and administrative entities. It is a vehicle for decision making regarding the economic, health, and social needs of community members under its jurisdiction (Roman, 2003). The people's council coordinates, controls, and monitors the delivery of health care and other services that originate at the national level. It promotes community participation in health care to assist the neighborhood in solving its health-care problems.

The Cuban health-care system brings together health professionals and community members from the national to the neighborhood level, which facilitates the utilization of existing resources for the health and well-being of community members. In doing so, the community is strengthened in the health arena, which is another aim of a socially ecologically oriented practice (Ungar, 2002).

PRINCIPLE 2: THE CENTRALITY OF COMMUNITY STAKEHOLDERS

A service-delivery system that is managed by community stakeholders, not bureaucracies, is the least likely to contribute to social disintegration.

Community stakeholders are integrated into the Cuban health-care system, and their participation is vital to health promotion and care at the neighborhood level. They include community-based grassroots organizations and political entities, including "mass organizations," which are involved in decision making about health care in the community. Community stakeholders coordinate with government entities, including people's councils, at the municipal and provincial levels, formulate health-care policy, and implement education and prevention programs in the community.

So-called mass organizations are entities at the local, regional, and national levels, created after the revolution, that are entrusted with a variety of public health, educational, and security functions within the community (Díaz-Briquets, 2002). Mass organizations that play a role in health care at the community level include the Federation of Cuban Women (FMC), the Committees for the Defense of the Revolution (CDRs), and in rural areas, the National Association of Small Farmers (ANAP). The FMC and the CDRs have been instrumental in building primary components of the Cuban health-care system since the beginning of the revolution (Barberia & Castro, 2002). The FMC organizes vaccination campaigns, conducts public education, and during economically difficult times has distributed vitamins to households and organized meetings to talk about cooking meals (Uriarte, in press). The FMC also helps to coordinate prenatal, maternal, and infant care. The ANAP has monitored and has organized educational campaigns concerning workplace safety. Senior citizen organizations in the community, known as grandparent circles (círculos de abuelos), assist health-care workers with geriatric medicine interventions.

Representatives of mass organizations meet with members of multidisciplinary primary-care teams composed of doctors, nurses, and allied health-care workers including sanitary workers, psychologists, epidemiologists, and social workers, who are responsible for reporting to one or more members of the local CDR. Primary teams focusing on maternal and infant care include representatives from the FMC (Waitzkin & Britt, 1989).

These community-based entities are directly linked to the health-care system, although they do not themselves directly manage that system. Mass organizations act as "pulleys" that carry up information and carry down initiatives pertaining to health and other matters. Thus, mass organizations have direct input into the health-care needs of neighborhood residents. Community members have the opportunity to discuss individual, family, and communitywide concerns about health directly with their community delegate (delegado), or the neighborhood representative they elect. The delegate in turn brings the concerns of his or her electorate to the meetings of the popular council and municipal assembly. Delegates report directly to the community on the issues they are expected to resolve at these assemblies (Uriarte, 2002). The most common reason for a delegate's inability to resolve an issue at the local level is that municipal leaders lack power and also control over the resources needed to correct various problems.

The participation of Cuban community stakeholders and health professionals in community health initiatives illustrates the importance of human capital in the Cuban health-care system. Perhaps equally relevant is social capital, or level of neighborhood connectedness. The government promotes social capital, or community connectedness, by fostering community members' sense of responsibility to work together with health professionals to improve the well-being of the neighborhood. Notions of social responsibility permeate all levels of Cuban society and are an essential element in the Cuban government's postrevolutionary ideology. Spiegel and colleagues (Spiegel, Bonet, Yassi, Mas, Tate, & Ibarra, 2001) note that in Cuba social capital may be a stronger predictor of health within the community than are individual-level determinants. They suggest there exists a high level of social capability to undertake collaborative activity at the local level to address collective needs, as was demonstrated by Cuba's collective effort to address the 2002–2003 dengue outbreak in Havana. This and subsequent dengue epidemics have triggered widespread mobilization, volunteer labor, and a high degree of cooperation and compliance.

PRINCIPLE 3: THE IMPORTANCE OF PUBLIC POLICY

Public policy is needed that expands the capacity of communities and their members to function on their own by providing the resources they need to sustain their well-being.

This principle from social ecology suggests that health and social problems should not be implemented on the basis of narrowly defined programmatic interventions. Rather, it is important to implement public policy that is aimed at eliminating the causes of health and social problems. This principle emphasizes the need for social responsibility by the wider society for the health and well-being of the local community while at the same time offering communities the resources they need to sustain their well-being.

The Cuban government's ability to provide communities with the resources they need to address their own challenges has been limited by economic challenges and scarce resources. In the face of these limitations, the government has attempted to maximize efficacy in the health arena by partnering with the local communities. This approach coincided with the growth of the so-called neighborhood movement in the 1990s, when the community became the central locus for new social development and prevention efforts and for delivering services to vulnerable groups (Dilla, 1999). The central government delegated to regional and local authorities and to mass organizations the responsibility of identifying at-risk individuals with special service needs and determining ways of meeting those needs. The Cuban constitution created the people's councils.

Government has partnered with local communities in many different ways to implement broad-based interventions at the national and local levels aimed at improving health outcomes for the Cuban people. These health outcomes have been achieved by the use of a variety of nonmedical determinants as noted earlier (education, housing, clean air and water, nutrition, and employment), by social mediators (social cohesion, income disparities, and other social structure inequalities), and by health service determinants (accessibility, universality, comprehensiveness, quality, horizontal integration, primary-care focus, integration across sectors, and health-promotion focus [Dresang et al., 2005]). For example, the prevalence of low-birth-weight babies born in Cuba began to increase in the early 1990s. The government then established a national program, which represented collaboration between the Ministry of Public Health (MINSAP) and local governments, to address the nutritional needs of at-risk pregnant women. These women are identified by family doctors, health officials, and members of mass organizations and connected to Maternity Homes (*Hogares Maternos*). The homes provide preventive care, education, social assistance, and recreation for pregnant women and their children (Uriarte, 2002).

The government uses a variety of methods for identifying community members at high risk for health problems. For example, Cuba has recently started social work schools for the rapid training of students. These schools have graduated thousands of social workers who live in the communities where they work and who assist community representatives, mass organizations, and neighborhood members to identify adolescents, women of child-bearing age, and older adults who are at risk for a variety of health and social problems (Strug, 2006).

The Social and Community Context of Health and Health Care in Cuba

Health in Cuba is viewed in a social context and from a public-health perspective rather than from a medical one, as typical in the United States. In the United States, conditions such as alcoholism, sadness and depression, and hyperactivity disorder in children are frequently viewed as medical problems requiring medication, whereas in Cuba these conditions are typically viewed as social problems and as concerns that require a public-health approach and social intervention at the community level.

The focus in Cuba on community participation in health matters, on primary health care in the community, and on the relevance of social context in health and illness, are consonant with the health principles that emerged at the historic 1978 World Health Organization's Alma-Ata International Conference on Primary Health Care (Pan American Health Organization, 2003). This meeting called for the protection of the health of people worldwide. The principles espoused at Alma-Ata, which Cuba has widely embraced and incorporated into its community-oriented health approach, include the following: (1) Health is a state of complete physical, mental, and social well-being, and not merely the absence of disease . . . whose realization requires the action of many other social and economic sectors in addition to the health sector; (2) People have the right and duty to participate individually and collectively in the planning and implementation of their health care; (3) Primary health care is essential health care . . . made universally accessible to individuals and families in the community through their full participation collectively in its planning and implementation; and, (4) Health relies . . . on health workers, including physicians, nurses, midwives, auxiliary and community workers as applicable, as well as traditional practitioners as needed, suitably trained socially and technically to work as a health team and to respond to the expressed health needs of the community.

Cuba's Health-Care System and Health Indicators

Cuba's universally accessible, free, community-oriented health-care system may contribute to the country's comparatively good health-care indicators (Oficina Nacional de Estadísticas, 2005; UNDP, 2007/2008). These indicators are in some instances, like the infant mortality rate (5.3 per 1,000 live births in Cuba versus 7 per 1,000 in the United States) or the rate of life expectancy at birth for both sexes (75 in Cuba versus 75.8 in the United States) comparable to those of the industrialized countries. In addition to attaining admirably low rates of infant mortality and high overall life expectancy, Cuba has eradicated a number of infectious diseases including polio and has significantly reduced cerebrovascular disease.

Cuba has managed these accomplishments in health despite its economic difficulties and a U.S. trade embargo that has been in effect for close to fifty years (Franco, Kennelly, Cooper, & Ordúñez-García, 2007). Cuba has only recently emerged from the economic disaster it experienced when the former Soviet Union, its primary trading partner, abandoned the country and removed its economic support in 1990 (Spiegel & Yassi, 2004). However, despite limited resources, the chance of a Cuban child dying at five years of age is 8 per 1,000 live births in Cuba, the same as in the United States (UNDP, 2008). Cooper and colleagues (Cooper, Kennelly, & Orduñez-García, 2006) state that some observers are skeptical of these Cuban health indicators, but they note that Cuba has published extensive mortality and morbidity data by cause since 1970 and that manipulating original counts and maintaining consistency across categories for political purposes would be very difficult.

The World Health Organization calculates Cuba's per capita health expenditure at $229 and more than $6,000 in the United States. Nevertheless, Cuba has more doctors per capita, one per 170 people, than the United States (one per 188). In addition to its current seventy thousand doctors, sixty-five thousand new students have enrolled in Cuban medical schools since 2004. Cuba ranks 28th in the world in life expectancy, just behind the United States. However, Cuba's spending per person on health care is about a quarter of the spending of the United States (Atlas of Global Inequality, 2007).

In 2003, Cuba spent 7.6 percent of its gross domestic product on its health-care system, or approximately 236 U.S. dollars per person. It has repaired and modernized many of its more than four hundred polyclinics throughout the country and greatly expanded its health labor force, in particular its family-doctor program, which is at the heart of the Cuban health-care system (Franco et al., 2007). It has greatly developed its bio-pharmaceutical industry, a necessary step because of the U.S. blockade that prevents Cuba from importing low-cost medicines from the United States and elsewhere.

Cuba is able to achieve impressive health indicators mentioned above because national health initiatives are facilitated through the integrated Cuban public-health system described earlier. Universal primary health care and neighborhood organizations play a primary role in mobilizing the local community to facilitate vaccine immunizations, to screen at-risk populations to control infectious disease, to help prevent outbreaks of dengue fever and other diseases (Franco et al., 2007), and to educate the community about health. Social connectedness at the neighborhood level may improve individual health. Cubans are highly informed when it comes to issues of health.

References

Atlas of Global Inequality. (2007). *Health care spending.* Retrieved December 31, 2007, from http://ucatlas.ucsc.edu/spend.php

Barberia, L., & Castro, A. (2002). *Seminar on the Cuban health system: Its evolution, accomplishments and challenges.* Retrieved October 12, 2007, from the David Rockefeller Center for Latin American Studies, Harvard University Web site: http://www.drclas.harvard.edu/publications/working_papers

Bookchin, M. (1982). *Toward an ecological society*. Montreal, Canada: Black Rose.

Cooper, R. S., Kennelly, J. F., & Ordúñez-García, P. (2006). Health in Cuba. *International Journal of Epidemiology*, *35*(4), 817–824.

Díaz-Briquets, S. (2002). The society and its environment. In R. A. Hudson (Ed.), *Cuba: A country study* (pp. 89–156). Library of Congress, Washington, DC.

Dilla, A. H. (1999). Cuba: Virtudes e infortunios de la sociedad civil. *Revista Mexicana de Sociología*, *61*(4), 129–148.

Dresang, L. T., Brebrick, L., Murray, D., Shallue, A., & Sullivan-Vedder, L. (2005). Family medicine in Cuba: Community-oriented primary care and complementary and alternative medicine. *The Journal of the American Board of Family Practice*, *18*, 297–303.

Franco, M., Kennelly, J. F., Cooper, F. S., & Ordúñez-García, P. (2007). Health in Cuba and the millennium development goals. *Revista Panamericana de Salud Publica*, *21*(4), 239–250.

Longlett, S. K., Kruse, J. E., & Wesley, R. M. (2001). Community-oriented primary care: Critical assessment and implications for resident education. *Journal of the American Board of Family Practice*, *14*, 141–147.

Naess, A. (1989). *Ecology, community, and lifestyle: Outline of an ecosophy*. David Rothenberg (Trans.). Cambridge, England: Cambridge University Press.

Oficina Nacional de Estadísticas. (1998–1999). *Anuario estadística de Cuba, 1996, 1997, 1999*. La Habana, Cuba: ONE.

Oficina Nacional de Estadísticas. (2005). *Anuario estadístico de Cuba 2005*. La Habana, Cuba: ONE.

Pan American Health Organization. (2003). Alma-Ata revisited. *The Magazine of the Pan American Health Organization*, *8*(2). http://www.paho.org/english/DD/PIN/Number17_article_4.htm

Pérez-Ávila, J. (2001). An overview of the Cuban health system with an emphasis on the role of primary health care and immunization. In L. Barberia & A. Castro, *Seminar on the Cuban health system: Its evolution, accomplishments and challenges* (pp. A9–12) (2002). Retrieved January 1, 2008, from David Rockefeller Center for Latin American Studies, Harvard University, http://www.medanthro.net/docs/castro_cuba.pdf

Roman, P. (2003). *People's power: Cuba's experience with representative government*. Lanham, MD: Rowman and Littlefield.

Spiegel J., Bonet M., Yassi, A., Mas, P., Tate, R., & Ibarra, A. (2001, October). *Social capital and health in Cuba: Case study of a community-based intervention program*. Paper presented at the 129th American Public Health Association Annual Meeting, Atlanta, Georgia.

Spiegel, J. M., & Yassi, A. (2004). Lessons from the margins of globalization. *Journal of Public Health Policy*, *25*(1), 85–110.

Strug, D. (2006). Community-oriented social work in Cuba: Government response to emerging social problems. *Social Work Education*, *25*(7), 749–762.

UNDP. (2007/2008). *Human development reports*. Retrieved May 19, 2009, from http://hdrstats.undp.org/en/countries/country_fact_sheets/cty_fs_CUB.html

Ungar, M. (2002). A deeper, more social ecological social work practice. *The Social Service Review*, *76*(3), 480–497.

Uriarte, M. (2002). *Cuba: Social policy at the crossroads: Maintaining priorities, transforming practice.* Boston: Oxfam America.

Uriarte, M. (in press). Rediscovering "lo local": Potential and limits of local capacity building in Havana. In A. Kapcia & A. Grey (Eds.), *Revolution and participation: The changing dynamics of Cuban civil society* (pp. 197–253). Gainesville, FL: University of Florida Press.

Waitzkin, H., & Britt, T. (1989, December). Changing the structure of medical discourse: Implications of cross-national comparisons. *Journal of Health and Social Behavior, 30,* 436–449.

Waller, J. (2002, Spring). Healing by primary intention. *Health Matters, 47*(2), 17. Retrieved January 1, 2007, from http://www.healthmatters.org.uk/issue47/primaryintention

CHAPTER THREE

Overview of the Cuban Health System

Julie M. Feinsilver

Both the 2008 U.S. presidential election campaign and Michael Moore's film *Sicko* provocatively raised the issue of comparative health-care systems. Whatever one thinks about either Michael Moore's vision of the U.S. and Cuban health-care systems or, for that matter, Cuba's overall policies, one thing is clear: Cuba has something that more and more people in the United States would like, namely, universal health care. This fact was raised the last time universal health care was a major political issue in the United States. In August 1994, the *Boston Globe* even ran a cartoon depicting a fictitious conversation between then President Bill Clinton and Fidel Castro. Clinton asks Fidel, "Why should I negotiate with you?" He goes on to say: "Cuba is a poor backward island. What do you have that a superpower could possibly want?" In the last frame, Fidel answers with a question: "Universal health care?" This cartoon recognizes a major achievement of the Cuban revolution, one that has remained elusive not only for U.S. citizens but also for much of the world's population.

The questions then arise as to how and why Cuba could and would develop a national health system, how has it evolved, and what role it plays in Cuba's domestic and international politics. This chapter will address these issues and provide some comparative data regarding the results of Cuba's efforts.

Cuba's Health Ideology: Health for All

Although most government leaders supported the World Health Organization's initiative of "Health for All by the Year 2000," few have paid more than lip service to this ideal or allocated adequate resources for its development. In Cuba, by contrast, the revolutionary government has had an overwhelming preoccupation with health from the outset (almost two decades before the WHO initiative) and has directed its efforts toward improving health both at home and abroad. The underlying philosophy has been that health is a basic human right and a responsibility of the state. Moreover, the Cuban approach to health is holistic (physical, mental, and social), and it links health to the material environment in which each person lives. Extraordinarily, and unlike any other government, the Cuban government considers health indicators, particularly the infant mortality rate and life expectancy at birth, to be measures of its effectiveness. As a result, the health of the population is a metaphor for the health of the body politic. This constantly focuses government attention on both health conditions and the determinants of health. This unusual concern for the health of the population has been politically beneficial because of its contribution to regime survival.[1]

Cuban health ideology posited that medicine alone would not improve the population's health. What was needed, according to this ideology, was a significant socioeconomic transformation to eliminate the problems of underdevelopment. Health-sector reform, therefore, was only one part of that larger societal transformation, which included universal free education, a guaranteed minimum food ration, very low-cost housing, and universal social security, among other things. The guiding principles for that reform were: (1) equality of access to services, (2) a holistic approach to health (which required interdisciplinary teams to implement programs), and (3) community participation in health initiatives. Equality of access refers to a myriad of factors including legal, economic, geographic, and cultural access to health care. Legally, the right to health and the state's obligation to provide services were enshrined in the Constitution. Economic access meant universal free

---

[1] For a full discussion of the ideology and organization of the Cuban health system; health education and popular participation; medical education and the distribution of personnel; biotechnology, biomedical research, and medical-pharmaceutical exports; Cuban medical diplomacy; and the symbolic and very real material benefits of Cuba's approach, see Julie M. Feinsilver, *Healing the Masses: Cuban Health Politics at Home and Abroad*, University of California Press, 1993. Although the statistical data are dated, the overall analysis has, as Dr. Peter Bourne indicated, "withstood the test of time." (Personal communication from Dr. Bourne, executive producer of *Salud! The Film*, November 13, 2006.)

services for all. Geographic access required a major change in the distribution of facilities and personnel to reach all citizens, no matter where they lived.

Cultural access meant a decrease in the social class and educational differences between physicians and their patients. This was done through open enrollment for medical education and by training and stationing doctors in their home provinces, to the extent feasible. Open enrollment was ideologically appealing, but also necessary owing to the exodus of approximately half of the country's doctors shortly after the triumph of the revolution. A holistic approach to health not only focuses on the patient as a whole person and not just a body part, but also integrates prevention, cure, and rehabilitation.

Popular participation was envisioned as a means of involving the public, through their community-based organizations (Committees for the Defense of the Revolution, Federation of Cuban Women, trade unions, student organizations), in the planning, administration, implementation, and monitoring of health-service delivery in conjunction with local-level health establishments. Despite the rhetoric and initial government desire, community participation primarily has meant implementation of health initiatives, and this has been done with great success. Nonetheless, popular participation has given the public an opportunity not only to take matters into their own hands and see that they could solve some of their own problems, but also it has given them an education in certain health matters.[2] This has been an important part of general government efforts to enhance individual and community self-reliance and a step toward community cohesion.

An International Dimension

From the initial days of the revolutionary government, Cuba's ideology also had an international dimension. It was considered Cuba's duty to help other nations less fortunate in an effort to repay a debt to humanity for support received from others during the revolution. Therefore, the provision of medical aid (medical diplomacy) to other developing countries has been a key element of Cuba's international relations since 1960, when the island first sent a medical brigade to assist Chile after an earthquake. Since then, Cuba has utilized medical diplomacy as a way of winning friends and influencing people, of capturing the hearts and minds of aid recipients. It is a means of gaining prestige and goodwill (symbolic capital), which can be translated into diplomatic support and trade or

---

[2] Feinsilver, *Healing the Masses*, pp. 28–29.

aid (material capital). It is a way of projecting Cuba's image abroad as increasingly more developed and technologically sophisticated, and this is important in Cuba's symbolic struggle as David versus the Goliath of the United States. Cuba's success in this endeavor has been recognized by the World Health Organization and other United Nations bodies, as well as by numerous governments, at least seventy of which have been direct beneficiaries of Cuba's largesse. It also has contributed to support for Cuba and rebuke of the United States in the United Nations General Assembly, where for sixteen consecutive years members voted overwhelmingly in favor of lifting the U.S. embargo of Cuba. In fact, only Israel, Palau, and the Marshall Islands have supported the U.S. position in recent years.[3] Since the rise of Hugo Chavez in Venezuela, Cuba's medical diplomacy has been bolstered by trade with and aid from Venezuela in a large-scale oil-for-doctors exchange. Recognizing the political and economic benefit to Cuba of its medical diplomacy program, the U.S. government recently has tried to thwart it by offering easy asylum to Cuban doctors providing medical aid in third world countries.[4]

Aspects of Cuba's medical-diplomacy program will be discussed in a later chapter. However, some understanding of the evolution of the Cuban health system is important for understanding (1) how Cuba was able to export both its health-care model through direct technical assistance and medical education of foreign students, and its medical professionals through the medical-diplomacy program; and (2) how Cuba has achieved critical health indices comparable to those of the United States.

Evolution of the Cuban Health System Since the Revolution

Ongoing reform has been a key characteristic of the Cuban health system. During each decade there has been a reassessment of progress and problems, and adjustments made accordingly. Health-care reform has responded to changing health, social, economic, and political priorities over the almost half century since the Cuban revolution. What follows is a brief discussion of those changes by decade.

---

[3] See http://secap480.un.org/

[4] See Julie M. Feinsilver, "La Diplomacia Médica Cubana: Cuando la Izquierda lo ha Hecho Bien [Cuban Medical Diplomacy: When the Left Has Got It Right]," *Foreign Affairs en Español* vol. 6, no. 4 (Oct–Dec. 2006): 81–94. The English version is available at http://www.coha.org/2006/10/30/cuban-medical-diplomacy-when-the-left-has-got-it-right/; Julie M. Feinsilver, "Médicos por Petróleo: Ls Diplomacia Médica Cubana Recibe una Pequeña Ayuda de Sus Amigos," *Nueva Sociedad* 216 (Julio–Agosto 2008):107–122. The English version is available at http://www.nuso.org/revista.php?n=216. For a detailed historical analysis, see Feinsilver, *Healing the Masses*, chapter 6: Cuban Medical Diplomacy, pp. 156–195.

Health Sector Reform in the 1960s: Establishment of a National Health System

To achieve universal health care, the Cuban revolutionary government began its health-sector reform almost immediately after taking power in 1959. This decision was based on three important factors: (1) the revolutionaries' experience of the abject poverty of much of the rural population and their provision of medical care for the population living in areas under their control during the revolutionary war; (2) the example of prerevolutionary mutual aid societies that provided prepaid (HMO-like) medical services to their members; and (3) the espousal of social medicine by progressive physicians in one of two prerevolutionary Cuban medical societies (the Cuban Medical Federation). All of these factors facilitated the decision by the new government to form the Rural Health Service in January 1960, thereby establishing medical care in the periphery, where little or none had previously existed. New medical school graduates were required to serve one year as staff in the Rural Health Service. Health centers were converted to polyclincs beginning in 1964, each serving a predefined geographic population of between twenty-five thousand and thirty thousand. These geographic areas were further subdivided into health sectors with one internist per five thousand adults, one OB/GYN for every three thousand to four thousand women over age fifteen, and one pediatrician for every two thousand to three thousand children under age fifteen. A nurse trained in the corresponding discipline completed each basic team. Services were standardized and norms and methods centrally dictated. By 1967, the government had radically restructured the three health subsystems (public, mutual aid societies, and private) into a regionalized and hierarchically organized national health system providing referrals from one level of care to the next and most importantly, universal coverage.[5]

Health System Reform in the 1970s: Medicine in the Community

Although decentralized medical education began in 1968, it did not truly take off in a national sense until the mid-1970s, with the official introduction of medicine in the community and the conduct of part of each student's medical education in the polyclinic. Medicine in the community was meant to be the ultimate realization of the ideological commitment to health as more than just the absence of disease. It deployed the medical teams from the polyclinic into the community to attend their

---

[5]   Feinsilver, *Healing the Masses*, pp. 26–37.

geographically defined populations in their homes, day-care centers, schools, and places of employment. Importantly, the medical teams would begin their work in the community by doing an in-depth diagnostic of health conditions and determinants of health of their respective populations; develop a database of information on morbidity, mortality, and immunizations; assess needs and resources available; and select at-risk population groups for targeted interventions. These diagnostics were to be updated and discussed by the medical staff and community representatives every two months, but this often was not the case. By 1978, there was an evident disconnect between theory and practice with regard to the expected benefits of the medicine in the community model, particularly disease prevention, a reduction in the use of hospital emergency rooms for primary care, and continuity of care.[6]

Health System Reform in the 1980s: Closer to Home: The Family Doctor and Nurse Program

The inability of the medicine in the community model to solve the problems stated above led to system reassessment and further decentralization to the block level. Fidel Castro himself designed the Family Doctor Program piloted in 1984 to further project the health system's resources into the community by putting a doctor and nurse team on every city block and sending them as well to the remotest communities. The job of these family medicine teams was (and still is) to aggressively investigate and monitor the health of the whole population, not just the infirm; promote wellness; detect risk factors; prevent and cure disease; and provide rehabilitation services. Because the morbidity and mortality structures had changed from diseases of poverty to diseases of development, greater attention to prevention and chronic degenerative disease management became imperative.

This new model of health-care attention provided a family-medicine team for every 120 to 150 families or about six hundred to seven hundred people. This family-medicine team was backed up by an extensive network of health facilities of increasing levels of technological sophistication, from the polyclinic to tertiary-care hospitals and research institutes, as well as emergent biotechnology and pharmaceutical industries to supply them. Family doctors' offices with living quarters for the doctors and nurses sprang up accordingly. Although the Ministry of Public Health (MINSAP) provides norms for this program, there is considerable flexibility as to how to conduct the work at hand and

---

[6] Feinsilver, *Healing the Masses*, pp. 37–40.

great encouragement to spend more time seeing people in their normal environment rather than in the family doctor's office. This is particularly important because the family doctor's tasks include such activities as health education to alter unhealthy lifestyles and the promotion of physical fitness, particularly among the elderly. Cuban plazas and parks now look like Chinese parks, with senior citizens doing tai chi every morning at eight under the watchful eye of family doctors. The family doctor also acts as a patient advocate for any patients referred to the next level(s) of care: the polyclinic and finally, the hospital. The fact that patients can be monitored closely means that every bed in Cuba is now potentially a hospital bed. Data for 2006 indicate that 99.7 percent of the country is covered by 33,221 family doctors working in 14,007 family doctors' offices. Only Holguin and Santiago de Cuba provinces have slightly less than 100 percent coverage.[7]

Based on the practices of some of the world's best medical schools, Cuban medical education was revised to produce the new type of medical professional required to meet growing domestic and international goals. This meant a qualitative improvement in medical education, a curriculum change to a biological-systems perspective as opposed to the traditional disciplinary focus, the creation of a specialization in comprehensive general medicine (family medicine), and an integrated teaching-patient care-research approach to community-based medical education. All medical students, with very few exceptions, are required to do a three-year residency in comprehensive general medicine first, even if they elect to do another residency later. Most family doctors complete their residencies while on the job where they conduct research on primary health-care issues, and attend seminars at the neighborhood polyclinic where they are on call once a week. Professors travel to groups of doctors located in remote areas, rather than the reverse as is the case elsewhere.[8]

Although the Family Doctor Program may be criticized as excessive medicalization, costly, and possibly a form of social control, data indicate that it also has had various beneficial effects. For example, the following benefits have been reported: decreased costs due to more effective prevention, which resulted in decreased hospitalizations, surgeries, and emergency room use; lower morbidity and less use of medication among the elderly; and overall better patient compliance. More important, the program has led to a considerable reduction in the infant mortality rate in rural areas, improved health indices, and greater patient

---

[7]   Cuadro 93. Médicos de la Familia y cobertura Según Provincias. 2006. Año anuario: 2006 Fuente: Registro de Profesionales de la Salud y Dirección Nacional de Estadística.
[8]   Feinsilver, *Healing the Masses*, pp. 117–118.

satisfaction (according to MINSAP survey data). The program also provides a sense of relief and security for patients as well as their families. This in turn leads to greater government legitimacy.[9] Whether the benefits of this program outweigh the costs, which are quite different in a society where the state controls the economy and the education system, remains to be determined.

Collateral Activities

At the same time that great emphasis was being placed on primary care, the government also made considerable investment in the expansion and upgrading of its hospital network and the chain of specialized and high-technology research institutes, including the development of significant biotechnology and pharmaceutical research and production capacity.[10] It also invested heavily in the mass production of physicians specifically for its medical-diplomacy programs.

Health System Adjustments in the 1990s: Response to Economic Crisis

Ongoing reform has been a key characteristic of the Cuban health system. During each decade there has been a reassessment of progress and problems, and adjustments made accordingly. The decade of the 1990s was no different. The dissolution of the Soviet Union and the Eastern Bloc led to what Cubans called the "special period." As trade relations collapsed at the outset of the decade, the economy went into a tailspin. For decades Cuba had relied on the international socialist division of labor and subsidized trade, or what Cubans call fair terms of trade. Suddenly, basic necessities were no longer available, or, if they were, it was only at world-market prices in convertible currency. This situation was exacerbated by the long-standing U.S. trade embargo, which continued to force Cuba to purchase supplies from much more distant countries, thereby greatly increasing transport costs. The Cuban government estimates that this decreased its purchasing power by between 20 and 30 percent.[11] What had been problematic all along, such as shortages of some medicines and disinfectants, among other things, reached crisis proportions during the so-called special period. Inputs for the medical

[9] Feinsilver, *Healing the Masses,* pp. 40–41, 44–47.
[10] Ibid., pp. 58–62 and chapter 5, "Biotechnology, Biomedical Research, and Medical-Pharmaceutical Exports," pp. 122–155.
[11] See http://www.dne.sld.cu/minsap/indice.htm (La Reforma del Sector de la Salud).

system, replacement parts for equipment, pharmaceutical ingredients, and infrastructure components all became scarce. At the same time, the food supply was also seriously affected, making the population more vulnerable to disease. This dire situation left MINSAP with only one real option, to develop a strategy to improve operational efficiency in an effort to ensure the sustainability of the system.

MINSAP's strategy, therefore, prioritized the further development or deepening and/or expansion of a series of measures already in effect, which were not necessarily originally conceived for the purpose of cost containment even though that was one of the results of their application. These measures are as follows: (1) health promotion and disease prevention, (2) traditional or natural-products medicine and alternative therapies, (3) decentralization, (4) community participation, and (5) epidemiological surveillance. For example, the increased emphasis on health promotion and disease prevention had been a priority for decades and one of the reasons for constant system reform. Greater use of natural-products medicines and alternative therapies such as acupuncture and ozone therapy also had begun in the 1970s, but new emphasis would be placed on their standardization, reliability, and ability to replace some allopathic treatments.

Decentralization too had begun much earlier with the administrative subordination of the municipal-level health facilities to the Municipal Assemblies of People's Power (local government), which was supposed to facilitate coordinated cross-sector activities, as well as community participation. However, the new approach adapts the international Healthy Cities modality. In Cuba, by 1998 almost half of the municipalities belonged to the National Network of Healthy Municipalities, which encourages healthy living activities in schools, workplaces, markets, penitentiaries, and cooperative centers. This effort further requires the community, both as individuals and as a group, to take greater responsibility for their individual and their community's health. Finally, as a result of the optical neuropathy epidemic of 1993, epidemiological-trend-analysis units were created to improve the existing surveillance system by providing early warnings of disease outbreaks.[12]

Moreover, in response to the problems of deterioration of many health facilities, the lack of management capacity in many of the health units, and patient dissatisfaction with service, MINSAP indicated that it would revitalize the hospitals' operational aspects (and downsize them because the large number of hospital beds were no longer needed), give the family doctors greater problem solving capacity and some material improvements, and increase coverage, access, and the quality of care. MINSAP also would seek external funding to bolster the work of state-

---

[12] Pan American Health Organization, *Health Situation of the Americas 2007*.

of-the-art research institutes and clinical facilities. Change was necessary, but it had to be done with efficiency.[13]

Public Health Financing and Expenditures

Despite the severe economic crisis, the Cuban government ratified two basic principles of its public health system that reflect its ideological stance that health is a basic human right and responsibility of the state. The government stated that the health system should continue both to be government financed and provide free universal coverage. Public health expenditures per capita had risen considerably over the years, but most particularly as the overall economic situation of the country deteriorated. By 2006, it had increased almost one hundred–fold since 1959 (321.79 pesos per capita versus 3.72) and threefold since 1993 (107.57), the worst year of the "special period."[14] Even in the midst of this dire crisis, the overall priority for the health sector is evidenced by ever-increasing budgetary allocations as percentage of the state budget, with the exception of 1991 when there was a slight decrease. Between 1994 and 2000, public health expenditures increased 59 percent, with wages comprising the largest item. Central government spending showed a downward trend versus municipal government spending as a result of decentralization and increased focus on primary care.[15] However, the crisis vastly diminished the convertible currency portion available and used for health-care financing, which from 1990 through 1996 fluctuated between one-third and one-half of the 1989 pre-crisis amount in U.S. dollars.[16] This left the system's infrastructure and equipment in dire condition, except that used for health tourism, and therefore was a source of hard currency to be reinvested into the ailing health-care system.

The Twenty-First-Century Health-System Changes: Greater Focus on Results

Economic recovery, some of which could be attributed to the deepening of Cuba's strategic alliance with Hugo Chavez's Venezuela, allowed the

---

[13]   Ibid.

[14]   Cuadro 87. Ejecución del Presupuesto y Gastos por Habitante 1959, 1960, 1965, 1970–2006. Año anuario: 2006 Fuente: Registros administrativos de la Dirección Nacional de Finanzas y Contabilidad. http://bvs.sld.cu

[15]   Ibid.

[16]   República de Cuba, Dirección Nacional de Estadística del Ministerio de Salud Pública, *Sistema Nacional de Salud Políticas, Estrategias y Programas*. La Habana, Cuba, Diciembre 1998. http://www.dne.sld.cu/minsap/indice.htm (La Reforma del Sector de la Salud).

Cuban government to begin to rebuild its broken health infrastructure. After a decade of abandonment, plans were drawn to rehabilitate the more than four hundred polyclinics islandwide as well as at least fifty tertiary-care institutions (hospitals and specialized institutes) and fully upgrade their technology. At the same time, approximately one-third of Cuban doctors went to Venezuela to provide health services in an oil-for-doctors exchange. Both the state of disrepair of facilities and the sometimes shortage of doctors in a country that has prided itself on having the highest rate of doctors per capita in the hemisphere (three times the number of doctors per capita in 2005 as the United States),[17] has led to considerable discontent among the beneficiaries of the system. To address some of these problems, Raúl Castro announced in March 2008 that the Family Doctor Program would be reorganized to achieve greater efficiency and provide greater access in the rural areas.

Over the decades, the government decentralized services until they were delivered on each city block in an effort to improve health outcomes (with the result of containing costs through prevention). Cuba's demographics had changed over time, so that the graying of the population had become an important issue by the twenty-first century. The services senior citizens require differ sharply from those of the young. Also, as MINSAP planners reassessed the system using evidence from their statistical databases and the comprehensive diagnostic of the health status of each community and subsector therein, it became clear that the population in different areas required some different services based on their epidemiological profile. As a result, the decision was made to make services flexible depending on local needs. To test this approach, a pilot program was established in a Havana polyclinic, which was given greater human and material resources for implementation. This flexible approach should not only contribute to the improvement of health outcomes, but also could reduce costs.

Although the Cuban government has tried to ameliorate the rural-urban and other disparities from the outset and has made considerable strides in this endeavor, some differences have remained. Recognition of continued inequalities in health led to the proposal for and design of a system to monitor equity not only in the delivery of health services, but also in health outcomes and in the determinants of health.[18] This is part of an increased emphasis on achieving results in terms of health outcomes (i.e., infant mortality, life expectancy, absence of disease,

---

[17] Pan American Health Organization (PAHO), *Health Situation in the Americas Basic Indicators 2007*, p. 4.

[18] Abelardo Ramírez Márquez and Cándido López Pardo, "A Monitoring System for Health Equity in Cuba," in *MEDICC Review* VII:9 (Nov./Dec. 2005). www.medicc.org

etc.), which always has been a priority, and not just outputs (such as the number of physician visits, vaccinations, clinical interventions, etc.). Outcomes, however, may depend as much or more on improved sanitation and nutrition, both of which deteriorated in the 1990s, than on increased and/or refocused health-service delivery. Greater equity in the determinants of health will have to be assessed in the coming years.

Flexibility and Responsiveness

Two important characteristics of the evolution of the Cuban health system are the system's flexibility and the rapidity with which it can adjust to changes in health needs, medical technology, and international good practices or to domestic and/or international economic or political exigencies. The key facilitating factors have been political will and a vision of the future in which the health of Cubans would compare favorably with that of the U.S. population, at least on key indicators. Certainly as compared with larger countries with more complex economies and polities, the ability to make substantial and often fundamental change to the health system every decade has been striking. Cuba has been quick to adopt and adapt international good practices and to lead in some, particularly those related to primary care. As the economy either deteriorated or improved at different times over the past fifty years, the system quickly responded with increased prevention and health promotion (to counter deterioration) or the expansion of facilities and extension of the use of higher technologies (in better times). Finally, the Cuban health system has responded to the government's domestic and international political needs by producing both good health outcomes as measured by key indicators and good relations with countries receiving Cuban medical aid as will be discussed below.

Looking Inward: Key Outcome Indicators

As mentioned at the outset of this chapter, the Cuban government uses key health indicators as a measure of the health of the body politic. These key indicators, the infant mortality rate and life expectancy at birth, are used as proxies for socioeconomic development because of the many and varied inputs in their composition. Cuba rates very highly on both indicators despite its economic difficulties. By 2006, Cuba had an infant mortality rate comparable to Canada's and slightly lower than that of the United States. Cuba's rate then was 5.3 per 1,000 live births, whereas in 1960 the rate was 60 per 1,000 live births. Over this period, there was a steady decline in the infant mortality rate, but not without occasional temporary increases, which were always reversed quickly. The biggest reduction occurred during the first decade of the revolution. The rate dropped to 38.7 per 1,000 live births between 1960 and 1970. Then by 1980 it was 19.6; in 1990, 10.7; and in 2000, the infant mortality rate had declined to 7.2 per 1,000 live births. Life expectancy at birth was 78.3 years in 2006 and also compared favorably with the United States.[19] See Table 3.1 for comparison of Cuba's health indicators with those of the United States as well as the other "C" countries of this hemisphere, all of which have been considered models of health-sector reform at one time or another. Table 3.2 shows life expectancy figures for "C" countries and the United States.

Tables 3.1 and 3.2 based on:

Pan American Health Organization (PAHO), *Health Situation of the Americas 2007* data for the five "C" countries of the Western Hemisphere (Canada, Chile, Colombia, Costa Rica, Cuba) and the United States demonstrate Cuba's success vis-à-vis the other regional countries noted for their health systems and/or health-sector reform plus the United States, with which the Cubans like to compare themselves.

Table 3.1   Physicians, nurses, dentists, and hospital beds per 1,000 population

	MDs/10,000 pop. c2005	Nurses	DDS	Hosp. Beds/1,000 pop. 2005
Cuba	63.4	3.8	9.5	4.9
Colombia	12.7	6.1	7.8	1.2
Costa Rica	20.0	15.3	6.5	1.3
Chile	9.3	4.3	1.8	2.3
Canada	19.1	77.6	5.8	3.4
U.S.	22.5	78.5	5.4	3.2

Source: p. 4.

Table 3.2   Life expectancy at birth, 2007

Cuba	78.3
Colombia	72.9
Costa Rica	78.8
Chile	78.6
Canada	80.7
U.S.	78.2

Source: p. 10 (note: other countries are also comparable to Cuba on life expectancy).

That the Cubans admit their shortfalls is evidenced by their publication of statistics that indicate fluctuations in the most-important health indices, particularly the infant mortality rate at birth and the under-five mortality rate. They also admit the periodic deterioration of various

---

[19]   República de Cuba, Ministerio de Salud Pública, *Anuario Estadistico 2006*, Cuadro 22. http://bvs.sld.cu and PAHO, *Health Situation 2007*, pp. 8 and 10.

morbidity and mortality rates subsequent to outbreaks of disease or economic straits leading to suboptimal nutrition and/or sanitation. Since the economic crisis of the 1990s, the infant mortality rate rose slightly in 1994, then began a decline until 2000, when it rose slightly again, then declined until 2005. The rate again began a downward slope in 2006, when it reached 5.3 per 1,000 live births, which would be enviable in the most-developed countries. The under-five mortality rate paralleled that of the infant mortality rate.[20]

Universal health care, of course, is a key contributor to the abovementioned health outcomes and is itself a major achievement of the Cuban revolution. By 1970, there was one doctor for every 1,393 inhabitants of the island. In 2006, there was one doctor for every 158 inhabitants;[21] Cuba's network of health facilities in 2006 included 473 polyclinics, 243 hospitals, 138 medical posts, 291 maternity homes, and 142 homes for the aged.[22] More important than numbers of physicians and medical facilities is the willingness to experiment, to assess the system's strengths and weaknesses, and to make evidence-based changes. The current system still may be overmedicalized and too costly for strict emulation, but it—or aspects of it—serve as a model for others to adapt to their own circumstances. In that regard, it has had traction with the World Health Organization as well as with Venezuela, which is implementing a large-scale program with the help of more than thirty thousand Cuban medical professionals.[23]

Community Participation: An Important Instrument of Change

Community participation contributed to Cuba's ability to produce better health indicators over time. Indeed, it was critical for the success of mass vaccination campaigns, rural and urban sanitation drives, mass screening of women for cervical cancer, the early detection of pregnancy and provision of prenatal care, blood and organ donations, and the dengue campaigns. Not only did community participation have a positive effect on health promotion and the reduction of disease with vastly expanded coverage of campaigns, but also it led to quicker and less costly results, community self-reliance, and social cohesion.[24] The

---

[20] PAHO, *Health Situation 2007*, pp. 8 and 10.

[21] Cuadro 92. Médicos y Estomatólogos. 1970, 1975, 1980, 1985, 1990–2006. Año anuario: 2006. http://bvs.sld.cu

[22] Cuadro 99. Unidades Según Tipo y Provincias. 2006. Año anuario: 2006. http://bvs.sld.cu

[23] Feinsilver, "La diplomacia médica cubana," *Foreign Affairs.*

[24] Feinsilver, *Healing the Masses*, pp. 64, 80, and 89.

political significance of social cohesion generated by community participation should not be underestimated.

Looking Outward: Medical Diplomacy

Over the past forty-eight years, Cuba's conduct of medical diplomacy
has improved the health of the less privileged in developing countries
while improving relations with their governments. By 2008, Cuban medical personnel were collaborating in seventy countries across the globe.
Consequently, Cuban medical aid has affected the lives of millions of
people in developing countries each year. And to make this effort more
sustainable, over the years, thousands of developing-country medical
personnel have received free education and training either in Cuba or in
their own countries by Cuban specialists engaged in on-the-job training
courses and/or medical schools outside of Cuba. Today, more than ten
thousand developing-country scholarship students are studying in
Cuban medical schools. Furthermore, Cuba has not missed a single
opportunity to offer and supply disaster relief assistance, irrespective of
whether or not Cuba had good relations with the government of the
country in question. This includes an offer to send more than a thousand doctors as well as medical supplies to the United States in the
immediate aftermath of Hurricane Katrina. Although the Bush administration chose not to accept the offer, the symbolism of this offer of help
by a small, developing country that has suffered almost half a century of
U.S. hostilities, including an economic embargo, is quite important.[25]

An old Japanese proverb suggests that "vision without action is a day-
dream. Action without vision is a nightmare." The success of the Cuban
health system lies in the combination of both vision and action (supported by political will). This has led to health-system adaptability and a
reasonably rapid response to changing circumstances, which, in turn,
have led to the successes of the Cuban health system at home and
abroad.

---

[25]   Feinsilver, "La diplomacia médica cubana," *Foreign Affairs.*

CHAPTER FOUR

INFOMED

Pedro Urra

Initiated in 1992 during the so-called special period in Cuba, and partially reactive to the fall of the Soviet bloc, INFOMED, Cuba's online medical information network was founded with its main office located in Havana. INFOMED was at first designed to interconnect medical schools and institutions across the country, with the ultimate goal being to improve population health, maintain accurate and updated demographic health statistics, and confront infectious and chronic diseases with programmatic expediency (Delgado & Gorry, 2008). The development of INFOMED was facilitated with generous funding from several sectors: the United Nations Development Program, the World Health Organization, the Pan American Health Organization, and UNICEF (Seror, 2006). As Cuba began to recover economically and was able to invest more in information technologies, INFOMED's service was expanded throughout the country (Urra, 2008). Since its inception, INFOMED and the use of information and communication technologies (ICT) has proliferated not only in Cuba but worldwide.

The current mission of INFOMED is to continue to develop and enhance an integrated network for access and management of information for health care, training, research, and health-care management systems, with the ultimate goal of improving the efficiency of the Cuban health-care system. In addition, as an electronic medium, INFOMED fosters communication within Cuba and internationally with the scientific community, without regard for physical location. Within Cuba, a national infrastructure connects the medical science faculties to the fourteen Cuban provinces, for electronic messaging and access to electronic products and services (Seror, 2006).

In 2007, the editors were able to meet with Pedro Urra, the director of the National Medical Sciences Information Center and INFOMED, at the INFOMED offices in Havana. Pedro Urra responded to several questions that were posed at the time. The questions and Urra's responses follow.

Q. *How do you see the connections between the community and INFOMED, in both directions, community-to-program and program-to-community?*

U. INFOMED is a network of persons and institutions that work together and collaborate to facilitate access to education and information for the purpose of improving the health of Cubans and other people of the world, through an in-depth and a creative use of information and communication technologies. If we are to define ourselves as a network, and in particular a social network, then ties with the community are essential for the very existence of this network. This means that we want to be an organization that does not limit itself to the instrumental dimension of information networks. The institutions that make up INFOMED maintain a community perspective, especially with regard to the network's health libraries, which are located within local communities. In the specific case of our national headquarters here, which houses the National Center for the Information on Medical Sciences and the National Medical Library, there presently exists a direct connection with the community in which INFOMED is geographically located. This has to do with our relationship to a grandparents' circle, or group of older persons that regularly meets on the grounds of our headquarters. We here at INFOMED interact a great deal with the members of this grandparents' circle. Also, a community-based tai chi group meets here, as do other groups concerned with cultural and health-promotion activities. A public institution like ours has social responsibilities to the community that surrounds it in addition to the responsibility of carrying out our institution's mission at the broader national level. It is for this reason that we have an employee whose job it is to systematically coordinate our relations with the community that surrounds us, and those community relationships are quite good. Our ten years of experience working with the community along these lines confirms that it is both necessary and fortifying for both our institution and for the community to maintain an open relationship with one another. It is our social responsibility to have such a relationship, and, besides, it is a learning experience that can help us improve ourselves as an organization.

In what ways does community medicine in Cuba benefit from the existence of INFOMED?
By being a network of national reach that is extended throughout the country, and by having an important base in primary health care, INFOMED is aligned with Cuban health strategies that place a priority on community medicine. Despite difficulties and limitations that we have to regularly confront, the national health system and the government have prioritized resources so that there is at least one health library with dedicated personnel in each of the 498 health areas of the country. In the great majority of these libraries, there are computers and a connection to INFOMED, collections of CDs, audiovisual media, and literature that guarantee a base of information to support health-care activities in that health area. There are still some rural areas where online communication is not possible, and in these zones we work with options such as CDs and print literature, but they remain part of the INFOMED network; their library personnel support the work of the doctors, nurses, and other health workers, as well as health workers at the local community level.

How does INFOMED reflect the values of the Cuban Revolution?
INFOMED is essentially a project of the revolution, for it exists to support the improvement of the health of the nation, and, considering the impressive presence of Cuban health workers all over the world, we could say it exists also to support via its information network the health of many other nations. It is a network meant to provide information and knowledge to achieve equity and justice in health care, to support men and women who fight for these principles, and in this sense it is a project that uses technology with a liberating vision and not simply an instrumental one.

Which aspects of INFOMED most inspire you personally and professionally?
I am inspired by the fact that INFOMED was started at a most difficult moment, the "special period," and it has been in existence now for fifteen years, and that it is an enterprise that encourages us and inspires optimism. It inspires me because it is a collective work that represents the best efforts of many of us. It has always been aligned with the best values of the Cuban Revolution. INFOMED exists within the tradition of liberation of the Cuban

Revolution. We have overcome difficulties, incomprehension, our own shortcomings, because on the professional level, improvement and innovation have been a permanent challenge, because it has been aligned with humility and in a critical posture with the best of world development, because it has been articulated with our reality and has always recognized itself as still imperfect.

Where would you like to see INFOMED go in the future?
Toward a network that is continually learning, that is enriching itself with the participation of its members, that is organizing itself and aligning itself more and more in an intelligent and sound way with its overall objectives and priorities, and that measures up to an ever-improving health-care system that is worthy of a great people like ours.

What do you think other countries can learn from INFOMED's experience, including the United States?
That information and communication technologies should not see themselves separate from the social, economic, and political contexts into which they are inserted, and the essential thing is that these technologies be used in intelligent and intentional ways and that what ought to drive any project are the social priorities and the active participation of the people involved. It is fundamental that there be agreement among those persons who participate in the work of communication and information technologies. Their input into the construction of the goals those technologies attempt to achieve is also fundamental. The use of information and communication technologies is a process that involves the responsibility and commitment of each of its participants, and it is a process to which participants need to be made accountable and they need to constantly assess what they want to achieve. This is a social and a political undertaking which, to the extent possible, should have as its goal to improve the health of the larger community. As I have heard said a number of times, in the same way that health is too important to leave only in the hands of doctors, an information network for health is too important to leave in the hands of information specialists, although of course doctors and information specialists are both important in the network.

What are the challenges that INFOMED has faced in the past and that you expect it will face in the future?
I think that the main challenges have come from the situation that we are still experiencing in Cuba on a daily basis as a result of

the particular conditions in which we find ourselves living, which of course include the constant and systematic aggression of the United States against Cuba, and the blockade of Cuba is the most obvious example. Other challenges include our own inadequacies and problems that are related to difficulties that exist in our own society, which make it difficult for us to advance further. These inadequacies encircle us and we have to make greater headway in dealing with them. I believe that we are in a crucial moment in the development of the revolution, in which the active participation of all of us is necessary to resolve these problems, and to deepen the revolution is the only guarantee we have of facing the future with security.

To what degree is INFOMED multidisciplinary and "intersectorial"? I believe that the program is, in its very essence, multidisciplinary and intersectorial because it is sustained by human and material resources from other institutions. As a network of persons and institutions with a shared purpose, INFOMED has since its inception been receptive to the participation of professionals from varied backgrounds and to the collaboration of institutions located throughout the island. In fact, the services and informational resources are the result of the work and knowledge of specialists from all areas of health and other areas, although I think that one of the aspects that can place the work on a better foundation is to keep working consciously in this direction. There remain many challenges to intersectorality that require the resolution of institutional problems, but there exists the political will to overcome them. But as I mentioned in the preceding answer, these are issues that we need to work through and resolve so that the full potential of the network can be established and we can really become a network that can learn from what everyone has to contribute.

References

Delgado, A., & Gorry, C. (2008). Cuba's national health strategy. *MEDICC Review, 10*(1), 6–8.

Seror, A. (2006). A case analysis of INFOMED: The Cuban national health care telecommunications network and portal. *Journal of Medical Internet Research*. Retrieved June 29, 2008, from http://www.jmir.org/2006/1/e1

Urra, P. (2008). Cuba & ICTs: Real crisis leads to virtual innovation. *MEDICC Review, 10*(1), 52.

INFOMED can be accessed in Spanish at: www.sid.cu

CHAPTER FIVE

Medical Education in Cuba

Enrique Beldarraín Chaple
Matthew Anderson

The roots of medical education in Cuba can be traced to the colonial period, when informal medical teaching was initiated by Spanish monks. Formal medical instruction began when the University of Havana was organized in the 1720s. With the advent of the Cuban revolution in 1959, many Cuban physicians, including professors at the university's medical school, emigrated. This inaugurated a period of profound transformation in the methods and orientation of medical education. In the past fifty years, the evolution of Cuban medical education has been characterized by a major expansion in the number of medical schools and health-care workers, decentralization of health-care services and teaching, an orientation toward primary care with a central role given to family doctors and community medicine, and a close integration into the national health system. Cuba now plays a major international role in training health-care workers both at home and abroad. Cuban medical education reflects the broad values of prevention, community orientation, and a commitment to health equity that are characteristic of the national health-care system.

Historical Context

The origins of medical instruction in Cuba can be traced to the first years of the 18th century, when informal medical teaching was provided by monks of the Order of San Juan de Letrán at the Hospital of San Felipe and Santiago. Cuba did not yet have a university at this time, so the students were trained as *romancista* surgeons, a category of medical professional whose competence normally extended only to "external diseases." Formal medical education began in 1726 with the founding of the University of Havana; the University of Havana's medical school would remain Cuba's only medical school until 1961. The first medical students were three brothers from the Convent of San Juan de Letrán, and the medical school would remain under Catholic control until 1842 when it became a secular institution. Under the influence of the Catholic Church, teaching was largely scholastic and dogmatic; there was little experimentation, and cadavers were not dissected.

Surgical training did not start until the later part of the 18th century and suffered initially from a lack of professors. It was not until 1823 that a National Museum of Descriptive Anatomy was founded in Havana. Although this was not part of the medical school, it soon became an important resource for surgeons and obstetricians, evolving from a simple museum with wax figures into a teaching institution containing a dissection theater. This typified the development of medical education outside of the medical school, dominated as it was by the Church.

During the early and mid twentieth century, the medical school came under the influence of the United States, which occupied Cuba during the Spanish-American War. The curriculum focused on the diagnosis and treatment of the diseases of individual patients. Preventive medicine was neglected, as were social and community approaches to health. There was also a great imbalance in the distribution of physicians. According to the data of the National Medical Association, as of January 1959, Cuba had 6,300 doctors, 65 percent of whom worked in Havana.

The Revolution of 1959

The triumph of the Cuban Revolution in January of 1959 initiated an important period of transformation in public health and consequently medical education. The Ministry of Health and Charity was renamed the Ministry of Public Health, and Dr. Julio Martínez Paez, who had fought with the rebels, was placed at its head (Lenzer, 2008). Soon, a radical change in the culture of the Ministry occurred: work in preventive medicine began in earnest, and the first steps were taken that would culminate ten years later in the creation of a free, unified national health system. These transformations implied changes in medical education, not the least of which was a vast expansion of the health-care workforce. Unfortunately, such radical transformations were unacceptable to the traditional medical establishment. Consequently, these radical reforms met with marked resistance by the more conservative elements in the Cuban medical establishment, who were interested in maintaining medicine as a private, for-profit enterprise. The most dramatic tangible evidence of this resistance was the massive emigration of Cuban physicians in the years after 1959.

Crisis at the University of Havana

The birth of the new system took place at a time when the old system of medicine and medical education was already in crisis. The University of Havana, home of Cuba's only medical school, had been closed by decision of the University Council at the end of 1956. This decision resulted from student opposition to the policies of the dictator Fulgencio Batista y Zaldívar (who had taken power in 1952 by overthrowing then President Carlos Prío Socarrás). Student support for the guerrillas (led by Fidel Castro) who were fighting in the Sierra Maestra mountains led to a generalized confrontation with the dictator throughout Cuba's cities and most particularly in Havana. The brutal repression with which the student activism was met led to the closing of the university.

When the institution reopened its doors in January of 1959, a process of university reform began. The setting for this reform is captured in a document prepared by the Council of Higher Education (*Consejo Superior de Universidades*): "When the Revolution began its process of transformation on January 1, 1959 it was faced with a system of higher education that was disorganized, riddled with corruption and largely unsuited to the broad goals of renewing the country and developing it economically, politically and morally" (Alarcón de Quesada, 2002).

Many of the older professors at the medical school wanted nothing to do with the reform and retired in 1959 and the following years (Delgado García, 1988). The first years of the university reform also saw a process of political expulsions among the professors at the medical school. Some were fired because of their collaboration and ties to the Batista government, others for corruption.

At the medical school this situation came to a head at the end of 1960 when a proposal was made for joint governance of the school by both the students and the professors. This proposal had roots in Latin American university reform movements dating back to the beginning of the twentieth century. Most of the professors rejected the proposal, arguing that it was an attack on the university's autonomy. The government responded by either suspending or firing all professors who objected to the new plan. When all was said and done, of the original faculty of 161 professors teaching when the school closed in 1956, only 22 remained after the reform (J. L. Lopez Sanchez & G. Delgado García, personal communication, February 2004).

The resistance of the medical faculty was part of a larger movement of opposition to the revolution among the faculty at the University of Havana. Ricardo Alarcón, a law student and president of the Federation of University Students at the beginning of the sixties, remembers: "The university authorities basically caved into reactionary pressures. The Federation [of Students] was forced to assume responsibilities in the government of the university and actively collaborated with the patriotic teaching staff in developing reform plans, at the same time as [the Federation] was involved in other vital missions for the country" (Alarcón de Quesada, 2002 [translated from Spanish]). Thus, the conflicts at the medical school reflected broader conflicts both within the university and in Cuban society. Doctor Ricardo Alarcón de Quesada later held high positions within the Cuban government, as ambassador to the United Nations and chancellor and president of the National Assembly of Popular Power (Cuba's Parliament).

The medical faculty had to be rebuilt and new professors hired. This process permitted the incorporation of young, energetic, and highly motivated professors who were committed to the revolutionary process. They, in turn, facilitated the development of new health-care professionals who could serve in the novel health-care systems then being created.

Opposition and Crisis within the Existing Medical Profession

The majority of private physicians expressed their opposition to the revolutionary changes through the National Medical Association (Colegio Médico Nacional), one of the most conservative trade associations and an organization dominated by the wealthiest group of doctors. The years 1959 and 1960 saw intense debates among the membership of the association. In December of 1959, Dr. Oscar Fernandez Mell, a former commander of the rebel army, was elected president of the association. (He was later mayor of Havana and Cuban ambassador to Finland and England.) Seven years later, in April of 1966, the association dissolved itself, arguing that the existence of a separate doctors' union was no longer necessary in Cuba: "the defense of the rights of the doctor as a worker, as well as his and his family's protection against adversity due to disease, old age and death, are at the present time assured respectively under the National Union of Medical Workers and the Social Security Law, which protects all workers in the country" (*Tribuna Médica de Cuba*, 1966, pp. 27–28 [translated from Spanish]).

The changes in the National Medical Association took place during a time of massive emigration by health-care professionals. In the years following 1959, nearly all owners of clinics, laboratories, diagnostic radiology centers, and other types of ancillary services left the country. This exodus was especially intense after the nationalizations of September and October of 1960. This wave of emigration even affected a number of medical cooperatives and mutual aid societies. As a result, the majority of these establishments were transformed into Ministry of Health institutions.

The exodus of professionals in the first years of the revolution was extraordinary (Araujo & Rodríguez Gavaldá, 1966). In 1959, only forty-two Cuban doctors emigrated. The next year, 1960, 528 left the country, and in the following year 778. Between 1960 and 1965, it is estimated that 1,933 doctors left Cuba. By the mid-1960s, it is estimated only half of the doctors registered in 1959—roughly 3,000—remained in Cuba (Ramírez & Mesa, 2002). By contrast, in the years immediately prior to the revolution, the annual percentage of Cuban graduates who emigrated was 15.6 percent (Araujo & Rodríguez Gavaldá, 1966). This migration of health personnel was especially marked among specialists.

In December of 1961, new regulations attempted to stem the flow of doctors. Permission to emigrate was granted only after a several year's waiting period.

A parallel process was the progressive disappearance of many professional publications. Many of the journals published prior to 1959 ceased publishing either by decision of their editorial board or their owner. The only surviving publications were the *Cuban Journal of Pediatrics* (created in 1946), *Notebooks of Public Health History* (founded in 1950), and (at least until the first half of the 1960s) the *Medical Tribune*, journal of the National Medical Association.

Building a New Health-Care System

Paradoxically, the progressive self-destruction of the traditional medical establishment facilitated the reform of medical education, which started in January 1962. Young health-care professionals would be taught a new vision of their role in promoting the health of the nation. This new vision emphasized preventive care, primary care, reducing inequalities in access and outcome, as well as encouraging improvements in Cuba's medical research infrastructure and in the technical quality of health care.

Reform in education reflected the dramatic changes in Cuba's public health system in the period after 1962. These changes—motivated by Cuba's commitment to socialism—were a democratization and decentralization of education, the development of a rural health service, the creation of a free and universal health system focused on primary care and community medicine, the development of family medicine as a specialty, the integration of health care within the local political structures, and, more recently, a commitment to train health-care workers from other countries.

Expanding the Number of Health-Care Professionals

The Cuban medical system has been remarkably successful in terms of training health-care personnel. By 2005, there were more than 70,000 physicians working in Cuba; this contrasts with 6,300 in 1959. Overall, Cuba's health-care workforce is estimated at nearly 450,000 persons. In addition to these, there are more than 150,000 health-care students in Cuba, of whom about 22,000 are from other countries (see Table 5.1) (National Health Statistics Bureau, 2005).

Table 5.1 Health-Care Worker Trainees, 2005

Area	Cuban students	Non-Cuban students	Total
Medical students	25,728	21,863	47,591
Nursing students	35,483	120	35,603
Dental students	4,266	62	4,328
Allied health professions	67,472	776	68,248
Total	132,949	22,821	155,770

Figures for non-Cuban medical students are from 2006.
Source: Cuban Ministry of Public Health, available at http://www.medicc.org/publications/cuba_health_reports/cuba-health-data.php

In the early 1960s, new medical schools were formed and the deliberate decision was made to locate them outside of Havana. Medical schools opened in 1962 at the University of the East in Santiago de Cuba, and in 1966 at the Las Valles Central University in Santa Clara. The location of schools outside of Havana allowed local students access to medical education with the hopes that they would eventually practice in the areas where they were trained.

Training doctors, however, was seen as only one part of preparing a health-care workforce. The number of nursing schools was expanded from seven (1958) to thirteen (1968). In order to deal with the urgent need for health-care personnel, an auxiliary nurse program was created in 1960 and was eventually offered in fifty-eight schools. Training of nurse auxiliaries, however, ended in 1980, and existing auxiliaries were offered the opportunity to take additional training and become nurses.

Beginning in 1976, nursing schools began to be replaced by Polytechnic Health Institutes, which trained health-care personnel in twenty-four different specialties. In 2001, there were fifty-five of these institutions; sixteen of them included nursing studies. Over time, non-MD graduate programs were developed. By 1977, a master's level program in nursing (*Licenciatura*) was created (Delgado García, 1988). In 1989 to 1990, advanced degrees were offered in six additional fields: hygiene and epidemiology, physical therapy, physical rehabilitation, clinical laboratory techniques, x-ray, and ophthalmology.

By 2001, the health-care training system was composed of:

- 21 medical schools and their 290 associated training facilities

- 4 dental schools

- A national school of public health

- 29 Polytechnic Health Institutes

- 25 nursing schools

- A national center of technical improvement (CENAPET)

The results of this educational investment have been impressive. Between 1959 and 2000 Cuba trained more than 110,000 health professionals and 163,239 health technicians. Cuba currently counts 45,000 specialists in fifty-seven medical and dentistry specialties, along with 21,500 specialists in general medicine. This means Cuba has one doctor for each 174 inhabitants.

Decentralization of Health-Care Training

The medical-education system in Cuba has emphasized decentralization of teaching in order to promote geographical diversity in the health-care workforce. As mentioned above, the second and third medical schools were created, respectively, in Santiago de Cuba and Santa Clara. In 1976, this process took a leap forward when medical education was separated from the university structure and medical schools were created in several additional cities throughout Cuba. These new schools offered training in medicine, dentistry, and nursing. During the 1980s, Institutes of Advanced Medical Study were created in Havana, Santiago de Cuba, Santa Clara, and Camaguey. These facilities joined the twenty-one medical schools, four dental schools that were largely dispersed in the provinces, and the Institute of Military Medical Sciences (Delgado García, 1988).

Cuba is currently experimenting with the creation of "mini-medical schools" in local municipalities. Their purpose is to decentralize medical school training even further, with the goal of creating a more balanced health-care delivery system. Distance learning is being promoted with the creation of a Virtual Health University. New technologies have allowed education to be extended outside of the medical school setting into the workplace and even beyond the national borders of Cuba.

Adoption of a Family Practice Model

Beginning in 1984, Cuba experimented with a model in which primary health care was provided by a team composed of a family physician and family nurse. This program started with ten physicians at the Lawton Polyclinic in Havana and was eventually adopted throughout the country. Currently, 98 percent of Cubans are covered by some thirty thousand family doctors, thirty thousand family nurses, and four thousand professors (responsible for teaching students in the community clinics).

As currently organized, the nurse/physician pair provides integrated care to a defined population of six hundred to eight hundred people. The health-care team lives and works in the community, a situation that required either building new clinics or adapting existing facilities. Integrated care implies that the doctor is trained to study social and economic factors that influence the health of the population. The team's role includes improving the social context of health, a task that involves a broad role in health promotion and disease prevention.

In order to train clinicians in this model of community-oriented family practice, a new curriculum had to be developed with emphasis on subjects traditionally associated with public health, such as community assessment/intervention and disaster preparedness. A three-year specialist training program in integral general medicine was created for this purpose.

The *consultorios* (small offices) of family physicians have taken on an increasingly important role in medical education. Medical students train in the *consultorio* in close contact with the realities of the community. They learn how community conditions and risk factors can alter the presentation and natural history of diseases. They train in health promotion and disease prevention. Clinicians serve as their mentors and teachers. This type of educational activity is similar to that carried out in the Cuban polyclinics, where students train by working with specialists.

Academic Medicine

Beginning in the 1960s, medical research in Cuba was more tightly integrated into the work of the Ministry of Public Health. The goal was to link research more closely with sanitary needs of the country.

Several of the prerevolutionary research institutions disappeared. Among these were the Agustín Castellanos Foundation, the National Cardiology Institute, the National Tuberculosis Council Institute, and the National Institute of Nutrition. In 1959, the Carlos J. Finlay Institute was transformed into a School of Public Health. In 1965, the institute was moved to the old National Police Hospital and resumed work on research and development of biological products.

The only institute to survive from the prerevolutionary period was the Tropical Medicine Institute of the University of Havana. It was incorporated into the Ministry of Public Health in 1964 and renamed the Pedro Kouri Institute in honor of its founder, a renowned parasitologist.

In 1965, a National Center of Scientific Research was inaugurated. The center was created both to perform and to coordinate basic science investigation. A year later, eight Institutes of Medical Research were created; they would play an important role in the development of advanced biological technologies and in preparing medical specialists. Currently, Cuba has nine such institutes specializing in (1) oncology and radiobiology; (2) nephrology; (3) vascular diseases and vascular surgery; (4) neurology and neurosurgery; (5) gastroenterology; (6) cardiology and cardiovascular surgery; (7) endocrinology; (8) hematology, and (9) hygiene, epidemiology, and microbiology.

Parallel with these developments came new scientific and medical publications. The year 1960 saw the inaugural issue of the *Review of the Havana Psychiatric Hospital*. This was followed in 1962 by the appearance of the *Cuban Medical Review*, the *Cuban Surgical Review,* and the *Cuban Review of Obstetrics and Gynecology*. In 1963, the *Bulletin of Hygiene and Epidemiology* was inaugurated. All these publications were promoted by the Scientific Council of the Ministry of Public Health. In 1965, the National Center for Medical Sciences Information began the publication of a series entitled *Residency Topics*. These dealt with diverse specialty matters and greatly expanded access to specialized medical information, a need keenly felt by the growing number of medical students. In all, more than twenty volumes were published, each covering three to four topics (López Espinosa & Marqués García, 1991).

The National Medical Sciences Information Center then published *Laboratory Topics* and the *Journal of Reviews*. These publications summarized books and outstanding articles from the world medical literature. In this same vein, the National Center also published: *Current Information, Current Topics, Specialty Topics, Update, Medical Science*

Information, and *Direct Information. Current Information* collected journalistic information on medical advances from around the world; the other publications included recently published information about particular medical specialties (e.g., oncology) with an attempt to include a generalist's perspective. These printed materials supported the teaching and development of medical specialties.

More recently, the National Medical Sciences Information Center has been involved in the development of a national online network known as INFOMED (available at www.sld.cu), which provides access to a variety of Cuban medical publications (Séror, 2006). INFOMED also includes the Virtual Health Library, a Pan American Health Organization (PAHO)-sponsored project, one of whose components is to support medical education (Gorry, 2008).

Development of Medical Specialties

While residency programs existed in Cuba from the 1940s, the number of places was extremely limited. Postgraduate medical education began in earnest in 1962 with laws regulating medical specialties.

The Ministry of Health created National Specialty Groups including internal medicine, pediatrics, and surgery, which were led by experienced clinicians in each field. Among the tasks of these specialty groups was to unify diagnostic and treatment algorithms and to assure their consistent application throughout the country. The guidelines developed by the National Specialty Groups were published in the form of books. The first was *Norms of Gynecology and Obstetrics* in 1966. *Internal Medicine Norms, Surgery Norms,* and *Pediatric Norms* all followed. These manuals had inestimable value for doctors who had recently graduated and were assigned to the rural social medical service in remote and isolated locations. These publications were clear indications of the synergy that had developed between medical research, human resource formation, and the needs of the new Cuban health system.

In response to both scientific advances and changes in Cuban society, new medical specialties have arisen. Among them are traditional and natural medicine (TNM), intensive care and emergency medicine, and integral general dentistry (Portal, 2001).

Cuba's Role in Global Health-Care Training

One unique aspect of the Cuban system of health education has been its extensive involvement in international work. This has taken place on two fronts: the training in Cuba of foreign students, mainly from the

Third World; and the involvement of Cuban medical personnel in educational work overseas, including the creation of medical schools. This work began in the 1960s and was seen as part of Cuba's solidarity with Third World countries.

In 1963, systematic medical collaboration began with several developing countries that needed health-care professionals and technicians. Programs were created in Algeria and Vietnam (1963), Mali (1965), Brazzaville, Congo (1966), and Conakry, Guinea (1967). During the 1970s, medical solidarity was extended to countries in Africa, Asia, and Latin America.

In 1998, as a result of the destruction caused by hurricanes George and Mitch, governments in Central America and the Caribbean asked the international community for aid. Cuba responded immediately, expressing a desire to assist in the development of comprehensive health programs. By 2005, Cuban health programs operated in seven countries in the Americas, nineteen in Africa, and one in Asia. The need to provide personnel to work in these programs led to the creation of the Latin American Medical School (ELAM) in 1999.

Health Training Programs Overseas

During the 1970s, several medical schools were opened by Cuba in foreign countries. The first was in Southern Yemen in 1975 where Cuba constructed and equipped a medical school, staffing it with seven Cuban professors. The school opened with fifty-seven students (fifty-two of whom graduated in 1982), a number that eventually increased to four hundred. The faculty grew to encompass twenty-four Cuban professors and thirty-five Yemeni professors trained in Cuba.

In Ethiopia, Cuban professors worked with the University of Addis Ababa to create a medical school in Jinja. Cuba provided the first teachers in this school. Guinea-Bissau started its medical school with nineteen Cuban professors. Cuban professors have participated in the opening of medical schools in Guyana, Equatorial Guinea, and Gambia. In 2003, a Haitian medical school staffed by Cuban professors was opened with 120 students.

Training of Foreign Students in Cuba

In order to guarantee the sustainability of the integrated health-care programs it was developing overseas, the Cubans saw the need to prepare a qualified health-care workforce. Against this background, the Latin American Medical School (ELAM) was created in 1999. In 2007 it had an enrollment of 8,637 students from more than twenty countries. ELAM has graduated nearly 4,500 doctors (Giraldo, 2007), some from disadvantaged areas of the United States (Remen & Holoway, 2008). In Santiago, Cuba, a smaller Caribbean Medicine School was inaugurated for French-speaking students; in 2001, 254 Haitians and 51 Malians were enrolled (Morales, 2001).

The education provided at these schools reflects the values of the Cuban medical system. The goal of the schools is to train young doctors who will return to their native countries to work in their communities of origin, typically poor and rural. Consequently, students are chosen based upon their origin in poor and geographically isolated communities and their commitment to return to these communities.

In addition to these two specialized schools for foreign students, more than 1,800 additional foreign students are studying in the remainder of Cuba's medical schools. In 1999 to 2000, more than 4,500 students from ninety countries were studying medicine in Cuba (Morales, 2001).

Conclusion

In 1979, participants at the world community meeting at Alma-Ata made a broad commitment to "Health for All" by the year 2000, emphasizing the need to base health-care systems on primary care and to address the social determinants of health. Almost immediately after the Alma-Ata conference, these goals were declared "too ambitious, too costly and impractical" (Baum, 2007, p. 38) The commitment to a broad vision of health as a state of well-being has given way to underfunded international initiatives targeting medical interventions for specific diseases.

To a remarkable extent, Cuba has been able to make the Alma-Ata vision a reality (de la Torre, Marquez, Gutiérrez, López Pardo, & Rojas Ochoa, 2005). The medical education system simply reflects the values of that vision: decentralized, open to all, based on primary care, integrated into the community, and committed to equity. Thus, Cuban medical education stands as an example of what can be done, even in a country with limited resources. It directly challenges those who—on the basis of an apparently "rational" consideration of "practical" realities—tell us that another world in medicine is not possible.

References

Alarcón de Quesada, R. (2002). 40 aniversario de la Reforma Universitaria. *Revista Bimestre Cubana, 16,* 63.

Araujo, L., & Rodríguez Gavaldá, R. (1966). Migración de profesionales. *Tribuna Médica de Cuba, 26,* 14–27.

Baum, F. (2007). Health for all now! Reviving the spirit of Alma Ata in the twenty-first century: An introduction to the Alma Ata Declaration. *Social Medicine, 2,* 34–41.

Colegio Médico Nacional de Cuba (1966). Carta Internacional del Colegio Médico Nacional de Cuba. *Tribuna Médica de Cuba, 26,* 27–29.

Cuban Ministry of Public Health, available at http://www.medicc.org/publications/cuba_health_reports/cuba-health-data.ph

de la Torre, E., Marquez, M., Gutiérrez, J., López Pardo, C., & Rojas Ochoa, F. (2005). *Salud para todos sí es posible [Health for all: Yes, it's possible].* Havana: Sociedad Cubana de Salud Pública. Sección de Medicina Social.

Delgado García, G. (1988). Historia de la enseñanza médica superior en Cuba. *Cuadernos de Historia de la Salud Pública, 75,* 135–200.

Giraldo, G. (2007). Cuba's piece in the global health workforce puzzle. *MEDICC Review, 9,* 44–47.

Gorry, C. (2008). Cuba's virtual libraries: Knowledge sharing for the developing world. *MEDICC Review, 10,* 9–12.

Lenzer, J. (2008). Sergio del Valle Jimenez. *British Medical Journal, 336,* 162.

López Espinosa, J. A., & Marqués García, J. N. (1991). Apuntes para la historia del Centro Nacional de Información de Ciencias Médicas de la República de Cuba. *ACIMED, 9,* 88–99.

Morales, I. (2001). Formación de recursos humanos en salud para el tercer Mundo. estrategia de Cuba. In *Memorias del Encuentro Universidad Latinoamericana y Salud de la Población. Retos y desafíos para el siglo XXI* (p. 118). La Habana: MINSAP.

National Health Statistics Bureau (2005). *Annual health statistics report 2005.* Ciudad de la Habana: *Dirección Nacional de Estadística. MINSAP.*

Portal, J. A. (2001). Retos y desafíos para el postgrado en salud en Cuba. In *Memorias del encuentro Universidad Latinoamérica y Salud de la Población. Retos y desafíos para el siglo XX* (pp. 193–198).

Ramírez, A., & Mesa, G. (2002). El proceso de desarrollo del sistema nacional de salud en Cuba. *Revista Bimestre Cubana, 16,* 153.

Remen, R., & Holoway, L. (2008). A student perspective on ELAM and its educational program. *Social Medicine, 3.*

Séror, A. C. (2006). A case analysis of INFOMED: The Cuban national health care telecommunications network and portal. *Journal of Medical Internet Research, 8.*

CHAPTER SIX

Primary Medical Care in Cuba: A Historical Perspective

Enrique Beldarraín Chaple

At the present time, primary medical care in Cuba is conducted according to the model of the family doctor and nurse team, which attends to a local population of between six hundred and eight hundred persons. This plan mandates national coverage, which reaches even to the remotest geographical areas. Today these services extend to children's circles, schools, and major work centers.

This model of care has its theoretical basis in the ideas expressed at the conference of the World Health Organization (WHO) held in Alma-Ata in 1978, whose central theme was Health for All in the Year 2000. The event was dedicated to designing strategies and plans for different countries to offer to their populations (Tejada Rivero, 2003). In Section VI of the conference declaration, primary care is defined as ". . . the first level of contact of the individual, the family and the community with the national health system, which brings health care as close as possible to where the population lives and works and constitutes the first element of a permanent process of health care." It underlines the present importance of primary care as "the central function and the principal basis of the national health system"; Section VII.2 defines its modern direction as ". . . oriented towards the principal health problems of the community and [primary care] lends the corresponding preventive, curative, rehabilitative and health-promoting services" (Editorial, 1979).

Physician of the Week

The roots of primary care arose on the island in 1825, with the physician of the week model. Two physicians, one doctor and one surgeon, each week rotated without exception among all those registered in Havana. They were to treat, free of charge, the sick or injured poor of the town, some in their homes if necessary, or send them to charity hospitals (Delgado García, 1996).

The physician of the week team also served the function of forensic doctors; they inspected the hygienic conditions of public establishments and attended to the hygiene of foodstuffs that were sold in the city's businesses. From 1829 on, they had the added responsibility of the medical care of sick soldiers and mariners.

The names and addresses of the two weekly on-call physicians, with the dates on which they would occupy their shift, were announced in the official government newspaper of the colony, *Diario de La Habana*, appearing for the first time on March 4, 1825. Starting in July of 1837, they were announced also in the paper *Noticioso y Lucero* and a little later in *La Prensa*. On February 3, 1848, the *Diario de La Habana* became the official publication of the government, succeeding the *Gaceta de La Habana,* and the names of the physicians of the week continued to appear until this type of ambulatory medical assistance was eliminated. It is very interesting to note that the rotations for this service were rigorously complied with, and no doctor or surgeon could fail to carry out the duty, simultaneously maintaining his private practice.

This service underwent some changes related to epidemics and emergency situations and because of population growth and the expansion of the city. For example, during the cholera epidemic that occurred in Havana in 1833, which caused 8,253 deaths and triple that in the rest of the island (Beldarraín Chaple, 2005), a doctor was put in charge of home attendance to those affected, for each of the fifteen barrios within the city and outside it: three in the barrio of Guadalupe and two in each of San Lázaro, Horcón, and Jesús María. The physicians of the week continued as always for other medical emergencies (Martínez-Fortún, 1947–1958).

In July 1844, the city was divided into four districts for the purposes of improving ambulatory services. One district comprised central Havana and three districts were designated for the exterior, which included two barrios each: Guadalupe and Peñalver, Jesús María and Chávez, and Colón and San Lázaro. One doctor and one surgeon in each district and barrio were named weekly until March of 1848, when their on-duty times were extended for a month.

On January 27, 1829, the captain general ordered that the physicians of the week provide services to all army or navy officials who requested their service. In May 1853, a military doctor was named physician of the week, but on a monthly basis, for ambulatory care of military patients.

In July 1858, more districts were created; the district of central Havana was divided in two, which made five districts until February of 1859, when the fifth district was again divided in two, making the barrios of Horcón and Jesús del Monte independent. Thus beginning in that month, there were in Havana and its barrios twelve civil physicians on duty for the emergency care of poor patients, and to carry out their other duties, and one military physician to attend to the members of the armed forces (Martínez-Fortún, 1947–1958). The importance of this type of care in the early nineteenth century, at a time when Havana's poor and the Cuban population in general had no system of care to meet their basic needs, must be emphasized.

The Spanish colonial government had never until that time concerned itself with offering adequate medical attention to the population. The care of the sick fell to the Catholic Church with its charitable institutions and hospitals, and to the doctors with their private practices. The *Real Tribunal del Protomedicato* [the Royal Academy of the King's Physicians] limited its activities to organizing from a legal rather than a scientific standpoint the regulations of the medical and pharmaceutical professionals. In the case of an epidemic affecting the island, or of imminent attack, it dictated measures of control and regulation to be carried out by the Town Councils by prior agreement with the colonial governor.

These advances in medical attention to the needy, which began with the physician of the week, were possible because of pressures that began to be brought to bear on all sectors of colonial society by the members of the *Sociedad Patriótica de Amigos del País* [Patriotic Society of Friends of the Country], which arose in 1793. Because of this society, many health improvements were introduced at the start of the century: smallpox vaccine, cemetery burials, and the vaccinations of the slaves arriving to the island being among the most important. Enlightened, influential men of business (basically sugar growers), who already embodied what later became the national conscience, formed this society, and they demanded improvements of all types in national life.

This model of ambulatory medical attention improved over the years, but toward 1860 began to deteriorate; in July the military physician of the week was eliminated, since by then military health care was well organized. At the same time, the physicians of the week in the districts corresponding to the barrios of Horcón and Jesús del Monte ceased to be named. By royal decree of May 13, 1862, forensic doctors were named in the municipalities, and their regulation was approved, removing this important function from the physicians of the week (Vesa Fillart, 1888, p. 350).

Houses of Rescue

Starting in 1865, there were irregularities in filling the positions in the districts, which frequently had no physicians for several months. The situation worsened with the start of the Ten Years' War (1868–1878).

In 1873, the *Casas de Socorros* [Houses of Rescue] were created by the governor general's decree of August 24, 1871, and of October 24 of the same year (Delgado García, 1996, p. 152). The *Casas de Socorros* were part of the Municipal Health Service, which comprised ambulatory medical attention and house calls to poor patients, plus the services of forensics, autopsy, deputy inspector, and the office of food science.

However, it seems that some of the *Casas de Socorros* were functioning prior to 1871. In the public session of the *Real Academia de Ciencias Médicas, Físicas y Naturales* [The Royal Academy of Medical, Physical and Natural Sciences] in Havana on November 27, 1870, Dr. Antonio Mestre Domínguez, secretary of the academy, described the *Casas de Socorros* as one more step in the improvement of public assistance. He lamented that the *Casas de Socorros* had taken over the vaccination program and expressed concern that because there were *Casas*, there might be a public health concern. This subject was again discussed in the public session of January 22, 1871 (Delgado García, 1993, pp. 112–18).

In 1878, the director of the City Council of Havana and Dr. José Argumosa presented before that body a regulation for the Municipal Health Services, which included the obligations of the municipal doctors as well as of those of the *Casas de Socorros*. These regulations were approved at that time by the city council, as well as by the governor general on December 19, 1878. This was published in the *Gaceta de La Habana* later that month.

These regulations were later modified and again put into action on January 3, 1882, but three years later, on the suggestion of the council inspector of the Municipal Health Services of Havana, Dr. Serafín Sabucedo, a new series of regulations were discussed and approved. The new regulations, among other things, specified: "The *Casas de Socorros* must answer the need any injured or poor person has to be treated without any loss of time in public places or in private residences, giving first aid to the injured and carrying out the urgent surgical operations necessary, to enable the ill or injured to then be transported to home or hospital." In addition, "The *Casas de Socorros* will be served by two admitting doctors. In these establishments there will be, in addition, two medical practitioners and one servant, and the tools and medications necessary to aid the injured and ill." "House Attendance on Poor Patients will be entrusted to '*médicos de ascenso*' [doctors in training] who will visit in the home for those patients for whom it is impossible to go to an appointment, fulfilling therapeutic indications of the case and countersigning the prescriptions of those poor who are attended by doctors outside the *Servicio de Asistencia Domiciliaria* [Home Medical Service]" (Vesa Fillart, 1888, pp. 256–66).

In 1885, the thirty-six barrios of the city of Havana were grouped into five districts, and each was served by one *Casa de Socorros*, as well as another two districts in Arroyo Naranjo and in Puentes Grandes. They were the only ones available in the entire country (Mestre Domínguez, 1970, pp. 430–31; Mestre Domínguez, 1871, pp. 550–57).

At the end of the War of Independence (1895–1898), all that was available to attend to the population in Havana were the *Casas de Socorros*, the Home Medical Service to poor patients, the forensic service, the Municipal Hospital of Aldecoa, and a small disinfection team comprised of four men (Delgado García, 1996, pp. 33–36).

During the first years of the Republic (1902–1958), state ambulatory medical service again conformed to the model of the *Casas de Socorros*, but extended to the entire island, and services to the homes of poor patients remained in only a few *Casas de Socorros* of the city of Havana.

In the 1950s, the 126 municipalities of Cuba had *Casas de Socorros* in their principal population centers and in some others, the municipality of Nueva Paz, the present province of Havana, and another in Los Palos. These *Casas de Socorros* offered general practice, stomatology (now dentistry, oral surgery, etc.), treatment, and clinical laboratories.

The city of Havana was divided at that time into four districts, with a *Casa de Socorro* in each one: in the first district, on Corrales Street, Habana Vieja [Old Havana]; in the second district, on San Lázaro Street; in the third district, on Calzada del Cerro; and in the fourth, on Sixth Street of Vedado District. In all of these there were positions for medical students as practitioners. However, there were seven more in the barrios: Arroyo Apolo, Arroyo Naranjo, Casablanca, Los Pinos, Luyanó, Mantilla, and Muelle de Luz. Marianao had four, but cities of such importance as Santiago de Cuba, Camagüey, Santa Clara, and Matanzas had only one (Deulofeu Corominas, 1951).

The *Casas de Socorros* and the on-duty teams in the hospitals, as well as the clinics, which were principally for venereal diseases and tuberculosis, were the state institutions that offered primary medical care during the period of the Republic.

The Cuban School of Health Workers

During the early years of the Republic, the first half of the twentieth century, medical care was characterized by brilliant work in public health by a group of extraordinary public-health specialists who created a school known as the *Escuela Cubana de Sanitaristas* [Cuban School of

Health Workers]. This group included Dr. Carlos J. Finlay y Barrés, Juan Guiteras, and Arístides Agramonte, among others, who took Cuban health practice to very high levels. At that time, the first ministry of public health in the world, the Ministry of Health and Welfare (1909), was developed and began to function. It gave a strong impetus to the provision of medical care to the population, but by the mid-1920s, a group of the members of the *Escuela Cubana de Sanitaristas* had died and others had retired. By the 1930s, public health services had deteriorated and were insufficient since the population was growing, and in many towns and cities one *Casa de Socorros* was not enough.

Preventive Medicine in the Community

In the first years after the triumph of the Cuban Revolution of 1959, the old *Casas de Socorros* were converted to polyclinics with expanded consultation services and on-duty teams. In 1964, a new model for primary medical care was initiated, called *medicina integral preventivo-curativa* [preventive-curative integral medicine], whose health functions affected the people and the environment of a locality not to exceed thirty thousand inhabitants. Aleida Fernández, a polyclinic, was created as an experimental center in La Lisa, Marianao. When the results were analyzed and the experiment deemed a success, the scheme was extended to the entire country and was in effect for ten years.

Starting in 1959, the Cuban health system began to change its focus of action from curative to preventive medicine, developing from the earliest time preventive measures that were later complemented by measures to promote good health. This was on a par with societal changes relating to social safety and educational campaigns to raise the level of literacy of the population. This was a powerful incentive to the epidemiological campaigns begun in the 1960s, such as the polio and diphtheria vaccinations and the antimalaria campaign, among others, which accompanied improvements in the lives of the people. Following this general strategy, primary care was changed and developed with ever-increasing improvements.

Community medicine was conceived, designed, and tested experimentally in 1974 in the Alamar polyclinic. A year later it was extended to two more polyclinics in Havana City. This model, whose success led to its later implementation in the whole country, had as its basis the community polyclinic as the center of health services, caring for a population of from twenty-five thousand to thirty thousand inhabitants and was dependent on the *Poder Popular Municipal* [Municipal Authority of the People], although its operation was directed by the Ministry of Public Health.

These units functioned through the basic local programs: Programs of Care to Individuals (including integral care to children, women, and all adults, stomatological (oral health) care, and epidemiological inspection); Program of Care to the Environment (urban and rural hygiene, food hygiene, and workplace medicine); Program of Optimization of Services; Administrative Program; and Program of Education and Research. This system functioned for ten years.

In 1985, the country's national health system initiated a greater development of primary medical care with a new model—the family-doctor plan—that allocated health care to the entire population, divided into family groups totaling no more than seven hundred individuals per doctor. The new model was developed experimentally in 1984 with the placement of ten doctors in the Lawton polyclinic and subsequently generalized to the entire island.

The polyclinic was redesigned and transformed into a center of support for and control of the activities of the family doctor. Numerous medical specialties previously offered in the hospitals were incorporated into the polyclinics. Diagnostic, therapeutic, and rehabilitation resources made them into points of reference, support, and coordination for the work of the family doctor.

The family doctors are focused on studying economic and social factors and their influence on the state of the health of their patients, and raising that state through extensive work in health promotion and preventive medicine. The progressive development of this health system necessitated the new construction of doctors' offices or the adaptation of sites to serve this system.

The positive evolution of the plan involved a concomitant emergence of the specialty of integral general medicine. Accordingly, family doctors can accomplish these studies and later continue their practice in their own medical offices, but with a higher technical qualification.

In each area of health, the doctors' offices have been divided into *Grupos Básicos de Trabajo* [basic work groups], which are attended by three basic specialists: an internist, a pediatrician, and a *ginecobstetra* [ob-gyn, or obstetrician-gynecologist], to whom are added a psychologist and, where possible, a social worker. These groups provide consultancy to the office doctors in addition to offering specialized care to the population served there. Since 1984, when the model of family doctor and nurse began, it has grown year by year and now comprises thirty thousand doctors, thirty-two thousand nurses, and four thousand professors, covering 98 percent of the population.

The objectives of this program are:

- Access by the public to health services;

- Development of healthy communities;

- Achievement of healthy behaviors and lifestyles; and

- Care of prioritized groups.

Primary care of the population is organized, continuous, and in a dynamic process of evaluation and planned holistic intervention with a clinical, epidemiological, and social focus on the health status of individuals and families. Its objectives are:

- To develop a process of continuous improvement of the health status of individuals and families;

- To raise the population's level of satisfaction with the health services offered by the system;

- To determine the health status of individuals and families;

- To promote healthy lifestyles in individuals and families;

- To identify and intervene in the risks, illnesses, and other dangers to individual and family health;

- To facilitate interdisciplinary intervention in individual and family health problems;

- To provide the necessary information about the individual and family health for the development of the analysis of the health situation;

- To conduct an analysis of the health situation; and

- To improve the efficiency of family medicine in the workplace. (Ministerio de Salud Pública, 1998)

This level of care is carried out through preparation of individual and family registries and the periodic evaluation of individual and family health. The evaluation of family health involves:

- The most rigorous application of clinical methodology to family medicine;

- The evaluation of epidemiological indicators of risks, harm, and disability, according to age and sex;

- The evaluation of the individual's perception of family function; and

- The family health situation of the individual. (Ministerio de Salud Pública, 1998)

When the population of each medical office is allocated for the first time, it is evaluated and classified into groups:

Group I.   Apparently healthy individuals

Group II.   Individuals at risk

Group III. Sick individuals

Group IV.   Individuals with deficiencies and disability

This classification is not static; individuals may pass from one group to another depending on the risks or health problems they present and on the actions taken by the doctors, hence the necessity of evaluating individuals periodically.

The most important duty of a family doctor and nurse is to assess a situation and determine what actions and measures are needed. Moreover, a study is undertaken in each medical office every year that results in a basic document that governs the action of the doctor in his or her community. It is a continuous process of identification and prioritization of health problems and of elaborating a plan of action to improve the health situation of the community.

Objectives include involving the community through consensus and negotiation, so that community members genuinely participate in the identification and prioritization of their health problems and in the evaluation of a plan of action that answers the perceived and real needs of the people. Social and community participation in the solution of health problems is a process inherent to health and its development. Community members and health providers actively participate in the identification of the problems and in the actions taken to achieve the well-being of the population. The fundamental objectives are:

- To improve the quality of life of the population;

- To contribute to sustainable human and local development; and

- To identify and solve problems in an integral way with the concurrence of the different social actors. (Ministerio de Salud Pública, 1998)

This community participation is of inestimable help to the work of the family doctor, particularly for the identification of risks and the work of preventive medicine and health promotion.

The Cuban health system was developed under a social concept of health that at present includes much more than the absence of illness. It overcomes the limits of the individual and includes a person's relationship and interaction with his or her environment. Health is a state of physical, mental, and social well-being. It is also designed to enhance the development of potential in every individual and to help them best function in and adapt to their environment.

In 1978, the WHO conference at Alma-Ata devised strategies for the development of primary care and to reach the goal of Health for All in 2000. Cuba reached these goals in 1983. Since the 1959 revolution, Cuba designed and attained the development of its national health system with the fundamental principles that would later permit the results advanced many years later in Alma-Ata. That is why it was not difficult for Cuba to reach its fundamental objectives so soon after the conference, since the philosophy implicit in all stages of the reform was equity, for all Cubans to have the same opportunity to access health services. This made it possible to take medical services to outlying and inaccessible places with the design and initiation of the Rural Health Service. The strategy of primary medical care was initiated, with logical modifications as the system was perfected and the objective and material conditions changed.

References

Beldarraín Chaple, E. (2005). *La medicina en Cuba. Historia y publicaciones*. La Habana: Ecimed.

Delgado García, G. (1993). El cólera morbo asiático en Cuba y otros ensayos. *Cuadernos de Historia de la Salud Pública, 78*, 112–118.

Delgado García, G. (1996). Conferencias sobre la historia de la Salud Pública en Cuba. *Cuadernos de Historia de la Salud Pública, 81*.

Deulofeu Corominas, M. (1951). *Instituciones médico-sanitarias de Cuba*. La Habana: Colegio Médico Nacional.

Martínez-Fortún, J. A. (1947–1958). *Cronología médica cubana. Contribución al estudio de la historia de la medicina*. La Habana: Estarcida.

Mestre Domínguez, A. (1870). Las Casas de Socorro y su importancia para la vacuna. *Anales de la Real Academia Ciencias Médicas, Físicas y Naturales de La Habana, 6*, 430–431.

Mestre Domínguez, A. (1871). Las Casas de Socorro y su importancia para la vacuna. *Anales de la Real Academia de Ciencias Médicas, Físicas y Naturales de La Habana, 7*, 550–557.

Ministerio de Salud Pública (1998). Programa de trabajo del médico y la enfermera de la familia. *El Policlínico y el Hospital.* La Habana: MINSAP.

S/A. (1979). La conferencia internacional sobre atención primaria. Declaración de Alma-Atá. Editorial. *Revista Cubana de Administración de Salud,* 5(2), 177–180.

Tejada Rivero, D. (2003). Alma-Atá: 25 años después. *Perspectivas de salud,* 8(2), 2–7.

Vesa Fillart, A. (1888). *Manual de legislación sanitaria de la Isla de Cuba y de todas las Reales Órdenes y demás disposiciones relativas a la misma con algunas de la península, que pueden considerarse como supletorias.* T 1. La Habana: Imprenta La Lealtad.

PART II

Health-Care
Interventions

CHAPTER SEVEN

Breast Cancer in Cuba

"Think of it as a stone in the road"

Joan Beder

Overview of Cancer in Cuba

As in most countries in Latin America, the cancer statistics in Cuba continue to rise. The statistics tracking by Cuban public-health authorities continues to show cancer's rise as a cause of death and years of potential life lost. They note that malignant tumors are now the leading cause of death in some provinces and the number-two cause of death nationally behind cardiovascular diseases. This trend has been rising steadily for the last twenty years (Gorry & Reed, 2007). Data from the Ministry of Public Health's statistical yearbook show that in 2002 cancer claimed 17,490 lives in Cuba, which then had a population of approximately eleven million, accounting for 23 percent of all deaths in that year.

Since the 1960s, the Ministry of Public Health has made efforts to control cancer: in 1964, the National Cancer Registry was created; in 1969, a program was implemented to expedite diagnosis for cervical-uterine cancer; treatment and diagnosis guidelines were established in 1978 and 1981; and the National Cancer Registry was computerized in 1986.

Also, in 1986, the Ministry of Public Health created the National Program to Reduce Cancer Mortality based on the experiences and recommendations of the World Health Organization. This program consolidated various cancer activities and began several new initiatives. In 1992, this program was renamed the National Cancer Control Program and had two primary objectives: lower mortality and incidence rates, and increased patient survival and survivors' quality of life (Rodríguez, 2003).

While organizationally these programs and efforts were well conceived, there was profound difficulty in implementation because of the economic hardship created by the ongoing impact of the United States embargo against Cuba, imposed in 1961, and the collapse of the socialist bloc from 1989 to 1990. When the socialist bloc crumbled, it initiated a time known as the "special period" in Cuba, which lasted for a decade. During the special period, the majority of foreign aid vanished, adversely affecting the health system's ability to monitor, control, and manage chronic diseases such as cancer. Before the special period, the Cuban health-care system had access to raw materials needed to manufacture pharmaceutical products and medical equipment from Western Europe. During the special period, however, Cuban physicians had to cope with a lack of critically needed medicines, diagnostic tools, vaccines, and medical equipment that had previously been available for the cancer effort (Barry, 2000). As Cuba has regained its footing, recovered from the special period, and found new resources with which to address medical concerns, attention has been refocused on cancer and other diseases.

In 2007, Dr. Teresa Romero-Pérez became the director of Cuba's new National Cancer Control Unit. The newly formed unit attempts to bring under one coordinating agency all cancer control activities, and harness all the resources—human, financial, technological—needed to address the particular cancer needs of each locale in the country. Dr. Romero-Pérez has created an aggressive four-pronged program to:

• Coordinate all centers throughout the country to establish the Cancer Observatory;

• Pilot cancer control and coordination programs in thirty polyclinics in Havana City, eventually extending them throughout the country;

• Share knowledge from pilot programs and extend the programs to the municipal level throughout Cuba; and

• Integrate non-health-care centers and institutions working in the field of cancer control (Gorry & Reed, 2007).

While Dr. Romero-Pérez acknowledges that cancer must be addressed with various strategies, she has stated that the most powerful tool in the control of cancer is not cutting-edge technology or a phalanx of specialists, but the Cuban family. Working together with their primary-care doctors and nurses, families are the first line of defense. She acknowledges that detection, prevention, and health promotion are crucial in the fight against cancer. But "... the cornerstone of the effort is the family, and the family is what brings our entire strategy together"(Gorry & Reed, 2007, p. 3). This theme of integration between the family and the health-care system is central to understanding the Cuban health-care model.

Breast Cancer in Cuba

Today, breast cancer is the world's second most frequent cause of cancer and the first cause among women (Álvarez, Garrote, Babié, Yí, & Jordán; 2003). More Cuban women between the ages of fifteen and sixty-four are killed by breast cancer than by heart attacks, accidents, suicides, or from HIV/AIDS (Acosta, 2005). According to the 2003 yearbook that lists statistics of all diseases in Cuba, 2,573 women were diagnosed with breast cancer with a rate of 45.8 per 100,000 inhabitants. The highest-risk group is women sixty years and older, which represents 39 percent of all the diagnosed breast cancer cases (Annual Health Statistics Yearbook, 2003). These statistics, while disturbing, are not different from those worldwide, where this pattern of incidence and mortality is repeated (i.e., breast cancer risk increases with age over time). In the United States, statistics on incidence in 2004 were 126.4 per 100,000 inhabitants (Ries et al., 2007). Initially, these numbers may seem misleading, as the number of cases in the United States appears much higher than in Cuba. These elevated numbers reflect the availability of and use of mammography, early-screening techniques, and more widespread breast self-examination procedures, which leads to earlier diagnosis (and higher numbers of those diagnosed) in the United States.

Part of the explanation for the consistent increase in breast cancer incidence in Cuba relates to the socioeconomic development of Latin American and Caribbean countries and the changes in women's reproductive life in the last fifty years. The fact that a large number of Cuban women either work or study and have become active in society over the last forty years owing to educational opportunities offered through the government has resulted in Cuban women having fewer children, later childbirth, and later menopause. In addition, dietary changes have occurred over the years, with more women eating fatty foods and meat. Another related factor is the impact of educational programs urging breast self-examination and the need for regular checkups. These programs have been enhanced over the years and information is regularly disseminated. All of these factors are acknowledged as indicators in breast cancer incidence (Robles & Galanis, 2002).

Attempts to enhance breast health promotion (breast self-exam, clinical exam by a physician, and use of mammography) and disease prevention have taken many forms in Cuba. However, fundamental to the Cuban experience is their conceptualization of health. In the Cuban model, great importance is attached to the contribution health makes to the life of individuals and entire communities. The orientation stresses looking beyond the loss of individual capacities caused by disease and highlights the direct relationship between health and the population's quality of life. Thus, breast cancer management and control has become a priority, with education and knowledge as a focal point in an effort to address the disease.

Countless studies have confirmed that a woman's knowledge of breast cancer, its signs and symptoms, has a beneficial impact on detection and outcome (Romero-Pérez, 1996). According to Dr. Romero-Pérez, Cuba's National Cancer Education Program (NCEP) for breast cancer control has adopted the Competence Model as its theoretical framework. This model attempts to socialize knowledge so that the population becomes involved and actively participates in the social production and management of their health. The population is educated toward risk-factor control, moved toward early diagnosis and treatment, thus reducing the time between detection and the seeking of medical attention (Romero-Pérez, 2003). The National Breast Cancer Control Program urges women to participate in their care by doing breast self-examination, visiting the family doctor yearly for a breast exam, and having periodic mammograms. Educational materials have been prepared by the National Breast Cancer Program for use in training health-care providers and volunteers, who go into the community to speak with women about risk factors, breast self-exam, and so on. The Federation of Cuban Women has been instrumental in supporting the National Breast Cancer Control Program (Romero-Pérez, 2003).

Breast Cancer Education—The Federation of Cuban Women

The Federation of Cuban Women (FMC) was founded in 1960 and has more than 4.5 million women members age fourteen and older. Its fundamental objective is to achieve full equality of possibilities and opportunities among women and men. It is a voluntary, nongovernmental organization, is self-financing through a minimal membership fee, and has an advisory role in all Cuban affairs relating to women, guaranteed by the Constitution. Its structure is based on more than seventy-six thousand grassroots chapters linked to the national level. Due in part to the efforts of the federation, Cuban women are involved in all aspects of national life, and their presence in education and health care has been prominent and decisive.

The FMC has social workers and health promoters within their ranks who work voluntarily throughout the country on a local/community level. These volunteers are trained to help women learn breast self-exam and risk factors for breast cancer. According to an interview with Dr. María Luisa Buch Bofill, the president of the Cuban Breast Cancer Control Program, "There are still women who prefer not to know the facts about breast cancer. . . . In general, the change [toward knowledge, care, and prevention] has been a substantial one in the last forty years. The Federation of Cuban Women has been a key element in this area . . ." (Buch Bofill, 2003, p. 4).

There are more than 175 Orientation Houses for Women and Families organized and supported by the FMC across the country. These are literally houses within the community, where women gather for classes in, for example, child care, breast self-exam, and gynecological concerns. It is where they can learn to knit or crochet, and where they can gather to be together. It is not unusual to see women sitting together on the porches of these houses talking or learning from a volunteer instructor. The impact of these gatherings cannot be overstated. These community-based venues serve as a basis from which breast cancer knowledge is disseminated and issues related to breast health and other areas of health are discussed.

Education and Detection of Breast Cancer in Cuba

It is axiomatic at this stage in our understanding of breast cancer to state that early detection is an essential aspect of treatment outcome for the patient with the disease. Ideally, women today are doing periodic breast self-exams, and, with early detection, living longer and reducing breast cancer mortality. However, Cuban women have been slow to adopt this practice; whether it is because the education is still relatively new and has not reached as many women as had been hoped or because as Dr. Bofill notes, that Cuban women have had very bad experiences and memories of breast cancer dating back to before the Cuban Revolution of 1959. In the years before health care was nationalized, there were very few specialists, women were diagnosed much later, and the treatment was minimal and of poor quality. Consequently, almost every woman who was diagnosed died. This legacy may explain why older women are skeptical about education and treatment. But, as noted above, the Federation of Cuban Women has been making strides in this area through both face-to-face contacts with women at the community level and through the media—television and radio—and handout materials. In addition, gains toward early detection are being made as many more women are educated, work, and are less isolated than before the revolution and may be more open to breast self-exam and the necessity of regular breast monitoring. The task of educating women about mammograms has been an ongoing priority of the National Cancer Program, and Dr. Teresa Romero-Pérez plans to expand the program as the director of Cuba's new National Cancer Control Unit (Gorry & Reed, 2007).

Equally axiomatic is the knowledge that mammography is a primary tool in detecting breast cancers. Until 1990 (before the socialist bloc withdrew) all Cuban women over thirty-five received mammograms on a regular basis at no cost. Now, typically a woman will have a mammogram every three years unless she is considered high risk for breast cancer (has had cancer before, has a direct family member with breast cancer). Even women at high risk sometimes will not have a mammogram on this schedule and will be examined once a year by their physician and have a yearly sonogram of their breasts (not nearly as reliable as a mammogram in detecting tumors).

The situation with mammograms is particularly troubling, as it has been acknowledged as the best and most reliable way to detect breast cancer. Several reasons have been put forth to explain the infrequent use of mammograms in Cuba: the U.S. embargo, lack of or poorly functioning equipment, and lack of education. Medical equipment and advanced technologies are the supply areas most dramatically affected by the embargo (Hauge, 2007). The embargo has seriously impacted the ability of the Cuban government to acquire both parts and mammogram film manufactured in the United States (considered the best and most reliable in the world). The embargo prevents the Eastman Kodak Company or any subsidiary from selling the U.S.-produced Mini-R film—a product specifically used in mammograms, as it exposes the woman to low levels of radiation—and while Cuba has attempted to buy the film elsewhere, it has proved expensive to import (American Association of World Health Report, 1997). In addition, the embargo means that Cuba cannot buy equipment or replacement parts from U.S. companies or their subsidiaries without a specific license from the U.S. government. This forces the Cuban government to purchase some of their technology from suppliers far away, increasing, by far, the cost (Barry, 2000).

Treatment of Breast Cancer

In order to detail the trajectory of patient treatment for breast cancer, an understanding of the design of the Cuban medical system is necessary. According to one authority, "In Cuba, medicine is public health and public health is medicine; there are no dividing lines, no turf fights, and no finger pointing" (Hauge, 2007, p. 40). Because of this dual emphasis, the Cuban primary-care system has created a qualitatively different way of improving and maintaining the health of the population. The success of the Cuban model logically leads to a questioning of the traditional medical model found in most countries, including the United States. The Cuban government oversees and provides medical care to more than eleven million Cubans through a network of hospitals, health centers (polyclinics), and family doctors. The system was designed to guarantee universal care through a well-developed decentralized system that delivers everything from basic preventive and primary care (family doctor and polyclinic), secondary care (hospitals), to expensive, sophisticated tertiary care (specialty institutes) (Pérez-Ávila, 2001). The Ministry of Public Health is the central authority charged with policy design and implementation of care. In 2005, there were 70,594 physicians and 33,769 family physicians, with 62.7 physicians and 79.5 nurses per 10,000 population, and 54,857 medical beds in Cuba (Annual Health Statistics, 2005).

Diagnosis

The point of entry to the health system is the Family Doctor Program, created in 1984, with a doctor and nurse at the neighborhood block level who are responsible for health maintenance for 150 families in their community. The *consultorios* (doctor's offices) staffed by the physician and nurse, both of whom live in the community they serve, are the basis for continual community-based patient care. Since the community they serve is the community they live in, they know its struggles, living conditions, sanitation, and so on. This holistic perspective allows for a deeper and more comprehensive view of patients and their condition. There is the expectation that the primary-care team will do home visits, and there is a strong emphasis on the living environment and sanitation (Hauge, 2007).

The polyclinic is the next level of primary care, which typically provides follow-up after patients have consulted their family physician. More than 470 polyclinics countrywide provide primary-care services in the 169 municipalities (Romero-Pérez, 2003). The polyclinics were established in 1963, specifically for ambulatory care, and are charged with directing all health activities for persons within their jurisdiction. The polyclinics are staffed with professional, technical, and auxiliary personnel, including social workers (Novas & Sacasas, 2000).

The secondary level of care, hospitals, provides specialized services for numerous illnesses and diseases. There are 248 general, clinical/surgical, pediatric, and other specialized hospitals that provide medical attention throughout Cuba's fourteen provinces (Gorry & Reed, 2007). Tertiary care is provided at the provincial level, with eleven institutes specializing in areas such as tropical medicine, cardiology, neurology, oncology, endocrinology, and rheumatology. Each institute has a medical facility and a specialized research area (Pérez-Ávila, 2001).

It would not be unreasonable to question whether there is a disparity between the urban and rural areas in terms of medical care. In a recent review of the Cuban health-care system, it was noted that Cuba's health-care reform strives to eliminate differences between regions and population groups. "Before the revolution people lived in appalling misery and died young of preventable diseases. Today, even if living conditions continue to be very basic in some areas, everyone has nearby access to a full set of primary care services." (Aitsiseimi, 2003, p. 600). As a commitment to enhance health care in rural areas, the medical schools make working in a rural area a compulsory part of postgraduate medical training.

Typically, in relation to breast cancer, a woman is diagnosed either at the family-doctor level or through the polyclinic where equipment is available to assess, through sonogram or mammography, whether there is a malignancy. Surgery is not performed at the polyclinic; the woman is sent to a specialty hospital for her surgery. Follow-up treatment will usually occur at the hospital level where oncologists and/or surgeons will monitor the patient.

Treatment

Medical management of breast cancer in Cuba is consistent with standard protocols used worldwide, with surgery, radiation, and chemotherapy seen as first-line treatment approaches (Santos, 2003). Optimal medical management, however, is not always realized. This is due, in part, to the effects of the U.S. embargo, which impacts the choice and availability of chemotherapy drugs and radiation treatments administered after surgery. The drugs are not always in sufficient supply, and supplies arrive at erratic intervals. Some drugs can be manufactured within Cuba, but the raw material needed to make them is also restricted by the embargo. While other sources exist for supplies and medications, it is acknowledged that the United States has the best and least expensive. Results from clinical trials held in the United States are not always accessible to Cuban physicians. Radiation therapy equipment manufactured by the United States is considered the best in the world, but because of the embargo, Cuba is forced to purchase equipment from non-U.S. sources, paying more (American Association for World Health Report, 1997). Alternative treatments developed by Cuban folk healers are also used frequently, including snake venom, herbal remedies, the poison of the blue scorpion, and the bark of the mango trees. Folk healers, especially in rural areas, are active in using and disseminating vaccines and formulas to address breast and other cancers (Acosta, 2005).

Culture as a Factor in Breast Cancer in Cuba

Culture is generally said to be comprised of shared ideas, meanings, and values. It is a social construction that is created, transmitted through generations, and includes patterns of behavior guided by common ideas, meanings, and values. Cultural explanatory models are a product of culture, as well as social and historical factors within a population. The explanatory models of lay individuals within medical situations relate to the way people conceptualize illness and help to give meaning and coherence to their physical condition. In addition, these models offer explanations about sickness and may guide one's behavior through illness; they may also explain the etiology, symptoms, and management of the illness. Sometimes the cultural explanatory model will reflect undesirable life experiences, past experiences with the medical system and illness, and medical experiences of others. These conceptions of illness are laden with emotional meaning. They are often in contrast to the medical explanation and management of the illness and may impact health and illness behavior in a negative way (Rajaram & Rashidi, 1998).

In a discussion about breast cancer for the Cuban woman, it is important to understand some of the cultural explanatory themes that define the breast cancer experience. They are expressed in attitudes toward family, self-care, fatalism, and social supports.

It is widely acknowledged that "In Latin cultures, a woman is expected to put her family before her own personal needs. She is expected to sacrifice her own sense of well-being for the welfare of her family" (González, Gallardo, & Bastani, 2005, p. 117). At the center of the family and as the family manager, she is the overseer of the family, with members heavily dependent on her. To avoid causing their family sadness and worry, many women will ignore their health concerns, which might mean delays in medical appointments, breast exams, and mammograms (Luquis & Cruz, 2006).

In terms of self-care and breast exams, Latinas/Cubans are taught to be modest, which provokes feelings of shame associated with performing breast self-exams and having examinations by male doctors (Ashing-Giwa, Padilla, Bohórquez, Tejero, & García, 2006). A common belief is that touching of the breasts is reserved for intimate partners (Rajaram & Rashidi, 1998). These cultural imperatives, while undergoing change in the last decades, still linger as a pervasive concern for many women. In addition, for those who have sustained mastectomy surgery (loss of their breast), sexuality and concepts of feminism are especially important concerns. The culture of machismo is strong in Cuba and sexuality, concerns about femininity, and body esteem, are important issues after surgery (Ashing-Giwa et al., 2006).

For many Latinas/Cubans, there is the belief that cancer is a death sentence and that individuals have done something to cause their cancer, whether through behavior or thought (Simon, 2006). Women holding this belief will understandably be reluctant to come forth with medical concerns, as they will be revealed through their illness as a "bad person" who has "done something wrong" to have gotten cancer. The fatalism of the belief that cancer equates to death has also inhibited women from seeking medical care, as there is the belief that they will die anyway.

Social networks are also a factor in the culture of the Latina/Cuban woman. It is through membership in her community that strong connections are formed and help-seeking behavior reinforced. Advice and information are freely exchanged. For many women, the "social experiences among members of the social network can change beliefs, values and priorities . . . Patients' positive and negative experiences with health care professionals are transmitted through the social network and become part of the cultural database of the community" (Rajaram & Rashidi, 1998, p. 761). As so many Cuban women gather in their community either through attendance at the houses established by the FMC or on a more ad hoc basis, membership in the community is a strong and consistent feature in the lives of Cuban women. This form of connectedness can work in a positive and/or negative manner for the breast cancer patient. The connectedness will enable extended caring and support; the impact of negative past experiences is also potentially reinforced in the community.

It is within this context—strong family presence and the centrality of the woman to family life, the reluctance to do breast self-exams because of issues of modesty and privacy, and the fatalism of cancer as a death sentence—that the Cuban woman experiences breast cancer. These cultural explanatory models underlie the diagnosis of breast cancer. It is the social network, the sense of community, which often will mediate these dynamic forces.

Grassroots Efforts of Breast Cancer Groups

A significant effort has been made by the Cuban National Cancer Program to stimulate and support community activism on behalf of breast cancer. One notable example of community activity is the annual Terry Fox Run for the Cure begun in 1998. Terry Fox, a Canadian, had his leg amputated because of cancer at the age of eighteen. In 1980, outfitted with a prosthetic leg, he began his Marathon of Hope, running twenty-six miles a day to raise awareness about cancer. He died after running 143 days. Terry Fox has become an identified symbol of courage and hope around the world. Since his death in 1980, many countries have sponsored annual events in his honor, and in 1998, Cuban athletic and health officials adopted the run as a way to encourage healthy practices and raise funds for the national Institute of Oncology and Radiotherapy. Since 2003, the Terry Fox Run Against Cancer has been held in Cuba in every municipality countrywide to publicize cancer's causes, effects, and best prevention measures (Gorry, 2005).

Specifically community-based activity on behalf of women with breast cancer has been initiated in Havana over the last decade. In the 1990s, several breast surgeons were becoming concerned about the emotional toll that breast surgery was having on their patients, and small, local support groups were begun that focused on adjustment, dealing with the family, and emotional aspects of the cancer experience. Much of the discussion in these groups focused on issues of sexuality, treatment, diet, nutrition, and self-esteem. The meetings were held monthly but were logistically challenging to get started, as the women came from all parts of the island, with transportation very difficult to arrange. Nevertheless, preliminary follow-up of many of the women showed the benefits of the group experience on issues of sexuality and self-esteem.

In the beginning of the breast cancer group initiative, many of the women had to learn to say the word "cancer" which for them, carried the connotation of death; the euphemism used was the woman had an "unfortunate illness." There was also the belief that the breast cancer was the result of a punishment for some behavior or thoughts. This mind-set about cancer is reminiscent of that in the United States in the 1950s, when the word "cancer" was not uttered (it was referred to as "the big C") and there was the unfortunate correlation between cancer and behavior. In the United States, that mind-set began changing with the so-called War on Cancer, begun in the 1970s during the presidency of Richard Nixon.

In 2003, eight Cuban women, all breast cancer survivors, and several physicians, joined together in Havana to initiate a broader group program for survivors and their families. Their orientation was biopsychosocial with a goal of elevating self-esteem and helping women go on with life after their diagnosis and treatment, while keeping a focus on the relationships within the family of the survivor. This emphasis resonates with the cultural explanatory model described above. The founding members were aware of the potential for depression and withdrawal of those diagnosed and treated for breast cancer. The early meetings of the women (considered board members) were held in hospitals or wherever they could find space. Plans to develop a countrywide program of support groups, hotline services, and educational programs were discussed.

The board members approached the Federation of Cuban Women, found a strong level of support for their program ideas, and were given space to hold their planning and support-group meetings. They began meeting once a month, with forty women forming the first open group. More women were contacted and the group continued to grow. The women put notices up on doors of the polyclinics, obtained radio time announcing their meetings, and had radio interviews with physicians. They began running television spots about group meetings, and printed educational items. A journalist made a documentary about the initial group of founding women, and it was aired on television. It was so popular that it was aired four times. Eventually, the large group that had formed was subdivided into several groups of ten to fifteen members. These groups meet regularly in the Orientation Houses operated by the FMC. Volunteers run the groups. Every month, all group members from each of the Orientation House venues are invited to gather for a Sunday afternoon meeting during which the family members of the survivors are present (the husbands of the women survivors prepare and serve lunch), the physicians who have worked with the women are invited, and the atmosphere is social and educational at the same time. Additional work of the volunteers includes hospital visits and home visits to women who have had surgery and are recovering. The group also participates in the Terry Fox Run Against Cancer (NB, personal communication, 2007).

By 2006, the group, now named *Alas por la Vida* (Wings for Life) was considering the initiation of a national helpline that would make telephone support available to any woman in need. New groups had begun outside the city and in the provinces. The group also sponsored a large art exhibit; forty-nine artists displayed their work, with each painting related to the theme of breast cancer. The group members are developing written materials on breast self-examination, urging the need for periodic examinations, which will be distributed throughout the country.

The Breast Cancer Experience—Survivors Speak

Several survivors—members of *Alas por la Vida*—were interviewed to detail their experience with breast cancer. The following is a portion of two of the interviews.

One of the women (M) was thirty-nine years old when she discovered a lump in her breast. She consulted her family doctor, who sent her to the local polyclinic where the physician diagnosed a 3 cm mass; a biopsy was performed as well as a sonogram. The results came a few days later, and she was hospitalized a few weeks after that for lumpectomy surgery (a small portion of the breast, at the site of the malignancy is removed rather than the entire breast); by then the lump was 5 cm. She was sent to the oncology hospital where she had surgery. She spent four days in the hospital and had outpatient chemotherapy and radiation there as well. She saw the oncologist every month. Certain that she was going to die, she grew depressed and anxious.

As she explained, she was very shy and a private person, and she felt very sorry for herself. When she was approached to join one of the support groups, she was hesitant, but after a few sessions she came to the realization that the worst had already happened and that she was happy to be alive. She commented: "I joined the group and met women who had had their surgery before mine. There was a lot of support, good learning, and I saw people who lived with their illness and I said, Why not me? So I learned that life did not stop with the surgery, that the surgery was a starting point to start living." When asked what her advice would be for a newly diagnosed person, she said, "I would tell the woman never to think that life was finished, it is the other way around, and always do what the doctor tells you to do. We all have our limitations but life goes on."

For another woman (N), diagnosed when she was forty-six, the experience was very difficult as there were other illnesses in her family occurring at the same time as her cancer. She had discovered a small mass in her breast, and because there had been several educational campaigns at that time, she went to the polyclinic. A biopsy was scheduled two days later, and two days after that she was hospitalized and surgery was performed. The diagnosis was a shock to her as she had felt well and had been working and fit. When the doctor told her of the diagnosis, she was astonished and terrified. She had a lumpectomy (only a small portion of the breast was removed at the site of the malignancy); a second surgery was performed to have her nodes studied for possible spread of the disease. (In the United States the practice is to do a lumpectomy/mastectomy and node removal all at the same time to spare the patient two different surgical procedures.) Typically, Cuban women stay in the hospital six or seven days. (In the United States, women are out of the hospital in some cases the same day, or after two or three days at the longest.)

For N, the time after the surgery was the worst of her life, as family illnesses were also getting more serious. Her surgery was followed by radiation and chemotherapy, which were very debilitating. When asked how she has been changed by the breast cancer experience she said: "I used to be a really happy person. I used to laugh a lot. Laughter was always on my lips. I never took things so seriously, as I never thought that death was so nearby. I have become a very sensitive and generous person." In terms of her follow-up care, N is considered high risk for breast cancer recurrence. As such she is entitled to yearly mammograms, but as she stated, she has a sonogram every year and while scheduled, she has not had a mammogram in more than three years. Her explanation is that the hospital does not have enough equipment and that they cannot get the parts for the machines, and when the machines are working, they are overloaded with new breast cancer cases. "There is intention but we don't have the resources."

As a founding member of *Alas por la Vida*, this interviewee feels that the group has changed her, but more important, she is pleased by the fact that the group has changed the lives of many women who would otherwise be going through this experience alone. Her personal philosophy has changed, and she feels that women who are facing breast cancer should think of it as "a stone in the road, you have to think that every morning the sun will rise, live deeply, and have joy as we have to continue living."

These two women, both survivors for several years, reflect an experience with a life-threatening illness from which they have recovered and been able to adjust their lives since diagnosis and treatment. Their experience is universal in that they have had to deal with and overcome the initial anguish and emotional turmoil wrought by their diagnosis. In the case of both M and N, the experience led to personal changes and activism to help others in their struggle. But unlike many women in other countries, both of these women were treated for their breast cancer at no cost. They were initially diagnosed at the primary-care level, and subsequent surgery and treatment were managed at the oncology hospital in Havana. They say that a cancer diagnosis can be life-altering, and for M and N it was, but it moved them from case to cause; their particular struggle led them to help others, and this is the guiding ethos behind *Alas por la Vida*. The care that they have received will surely prolong their lives, care given in the context of a political embargo that imposes many hardships. Nevertheless, they both are active and moving forces in their support group and demonstrate admirable courage and strength.

Conclusion

The experience of breast cancer for any woman, in any country, is profound. For the Cuban woman, the experience is complicated and enhanced at the same time by the medical care offered. Medical surveillance for breast cancer is available at multiple levels for women in Cuba, care is available, and treatment offered. Obstacles along the way include cultural beliefs (which have eased and are continuing to ease over the years), which impede seeking medical care, and availability of medications and adequate tools for diagnosis. The grassroots effort, in liaison with the Federation of Cuban Women, has impacted and will continue to impact the experience of breast cancer for many. The government initiatives and programs that are being established are dedicated to early diagnosis and support for the breast cancer patient. This is consistent with the community-based model of medical care in the country, with its focus on local intervention. By offering help to others—as shown in the statements of those interviewed—empowerment is achieved.

References

Acosta, D. (2005). Health-Cuba: Scientist, healers share aim of fighting cancer. Inter Press Service News Agency. Retrieved November 28, 2007, from: http://ips news.net/news.asp?Idnews=22293

Aitsiseimi, A. (2003). An analysis of the Cuban health system. *Public Health, 118*(8), 599–601.

Álvarez, Y., Garrote, L., Babié, P., Yí, M., & Jordán M. (2003). Breast cancer risks in Cuba. *MEDICC Review*, 2003. Retrieved December 16, 2007, from: www .medicc.org/publications/medicc_review/V/23/pages/mrinterviews.html

American Association for World Health Report. (1997). The impact of the US embargo on the health and nutrition in Cuba. Retrieved December 10, 2007, from: www.cubasolidarity.net/aawh.html

Annual Health Statistics. (2005). Cuba health data. MEDICC. Retrieved April 23, 2007, from: www.medicc.org/publications/cuba_health_reports/cuba-health-data.php

Annual Health Statistics Yearbook. (2003). Ministerio de Salud Pública, Direccion Nacional de Estadistica, La Habana.

Annual Health Statistics Yearbook. (2005). Ministerio de Salud Pública. Impact of cancer in women's population.

Ashing-Giwa, K., Padilla, G., Bohórquez, D., Tejero, J., & García, M. (2006). Understanding the breast cancer experience of Latina women. *Journal of Psychosocial Oncology, 24*(3), 19–52.

Barry, M. (2000). Effect of the U.S. embargo and economic decline on health in Cuba. *Annals of Internal Medicine, 132*(2), 151–154.

Buch Bofill, M. L. (2003). Prevention and treatment of breast cancer in Cuba. *MEDICC Review, Vol. V*(pp. 2–3). Retrieved December 16, 2007, from: www .medicc.org/publications/medicc_review/V/23/pages/mrinterviews.html

González, G., Gallardo, N., & Bastani, R. (2005). A pilot study to define social support among Spanish speaking women diagnosed with a breast abnormality suspicious for cancer: A brief research report. *Journal of Psychosocial Oncology, 23*(1), 109–120.

Gorry, C. (2005). Running for a cure: Terry Fox inspires Cuba. *MEDICC Review 7*(5), 32.

Gorry, C., & Reed, G. (2007). Turning the tide on cancer in Cuba. *Cuba Health Reports,* June 20. Retrieved January 2, 2008, from: www.medicc.org/cuba healthreports/chr-article.php

Hauge, S. (2007). Primary care in Cuba. *Einstein Journal of Biological Medicine, 23,* 37–42.

Luquis, R., & Cruz, V. (2006). Knowledge, attitudes, and perceptions about breast cancer and breast cancer screening among Hispanic women residing in south central Pennsylvania. *Journal of Community Health, 31*(1), 25–42.

Novas, J., & Sacasas, J. (2000). From municipal polyclinics to family doctor-and-nurse teams. *MEDICC Review, II*(3). Retrieved April 23, 2007, from: http://www.medicc.org/publications/medicc_reviewII/primary/cmframe.html

Pérez-Ávila, A. (2001). An overview of the Cuban health system with an emphasis on the role of primary health care and immunization. In L. Barberia & A. Castro (Eds.), *Seminar on the Cuban health system: Its evolution, accomplishments and challenges* (pp. A9–A12). Cambaridge, MA: Harvard University Press.

Rajaram, S., & Rashidi, A. (1998). Minority women and breast cancer screening: The role of cultural explanatory models. *Preventive Medicine, 27,* 757 764.

Ries, L. A. G., Melbert, D., Krapcho, M., Mariotto, A., Miller, B. A., Feuer, E. J., Clegg, L., Horner, M. J., Howlader, N., Eisner, M. P., Reichman, M., & Edwards, B. K. (Eds.). *SEER Cancer Statistics Review, 1975–2004,* National Cancer Institute. Bethesda, MD. http://seer.cancer.gov/csr/1975_2004/, based on November 2006 SEER data submission, posted to the SEER Web site, 2007.

Robles, S. C., & Galanis, E. (2002). Breast cancer in Latin America and the Caribbean. *Rev Panam Salud Publica, 11*(3), pp. 178–185.

Rodríguez, R. C. (2003). Cuba's National Cancer Control Program. *MEDICC Review, V*(pp. 2–3). Retrieved December 16, 2007, from: www.medicc.org/publications/medicc_review/V/23/pages/spotlighton.html

Romero-Pérez, T. (1996). Actualidad y proyecciones del Departamento de Control del Cáncer. *Rev Cubana de Oncología, 12*(2), 126–130.

Romero-Pérez, T. (2003). Education's role in the prevention of breast cancer in Cuba. *MEDICC Review V*(pp. 2–3). Retrieved December 16, 2007, from: www.medicc.org/publications/medicc_review/V/23/pages/spotlighton.html

Santos, A. (2003). Chemotherapy in breast cancer in Cuba. Retrieved December 16, 2007, from: www.medicc.org/publications/medicc_review/V/23/pages/mrinterviews.html

Simon, C. (2006). Breast cancer screening: Cultural beliefs and diverse populations. *Health and Social Work, 31*(1), 36–43.

CHAPTER EIGHT

History of the Cuban National Program for Chronic Kidney Disease

Robert Fortner

The kidneys are a pair of bean-shaped organs that lie near the spine in the middle of the back. Their main function is to filter waste products and excess water from the blood. In addition, the kidneys play a major role in regulating the composition of the blood, regulating blood pressure, maintaining the levels of certain minerals in the body, and producing certain hormones that have important functions in the body. Kidney (renal) disease has many causes and may result in permanent failure of the kidneys to perform. In the event of kidney failure, dialysis—the process of cleansing and regulating the blood through artificial means— may be initiated. A nephrologist manages the care of those with kidney disease. Kidney disease is present in all countries; the care of those with kidney disease in Cuba, similar to management of many diseases, is notable in many ways.

Cuba lies within a region (Latin America) that is comprised of thirty-four countries and more than seventy-six million inhabitants, of whom 40 percent live in poverty with no safety net. Hypertension and communicable disease are common risk factors for kidney disease, and the poor and near-poor alike have high incidences of obesity and diabetes, also factors in the disease. In much of the region, health-care facilities are scattered and often substandard, which is reflected in mortality outcomes. In contrast, Cuba, with more than eleven million inhabitants of similar ethnic heritage, while also resource poor, provides a comprehensive, free, prevention-focused health system with outcomes in infant and adult survival rates that match or exceed comparable statistics in the United States (Working together for health, 2006).

Nephrology in Cuba

The development of nephrology as a medical specialty in Cuba parallels that of other countries in which physicians, generally internists, undergo up to three years of additional training in diseases of the kidney. In the absence of trained nephrologists and with three new artificial kidney machines (see Glossary) available, Cuban internists, following the 1959 Cuban Revolution, initiated an effort to provide artificial kidney treatments (dialysis) to patients with acute renal failure (ARF) (see Glossary). Though they lacked the specialist training, as dialysis was not available prior to the revolution, they succeeded in developing the treatment capability in three areas of Cuba: Santiago de Cuba (eastern Cuba), Villa Clara Province in the center, and in Havana. As these capabilities evolved, the leaders recognized the need for trained specialists, clinical research, and treatment to prevent acute renal failure.

Importantly for Cuba, physicians who subsequently completed the training became the scientific and clinical base of the remarkable specialty program that exists in Cuba today. They participated in the creation and staffing of the National Institute of Nephrology in Havana and the first hospitals with dialysis capability. Established by the government through the Ministry of Public Health, the nephrology institute is one of eight specialty clinical and research entities that provide leadership and direction in their respective fields. By 1969, chronic dialysis for growing numbers of patients with end-stage renal disease (ESRD) (see Glossary) was underway, and in 1970, the first cadaver transplant was performed. In response to a 2002 Castro health directive (Chronic kidney disease, 2006), expansions were mandated to meet the growing demand and to reduce travel time for patients and families. Thus, in 2002, dialysis facilities, initially confined to the larger hospitals, were expanded and new centers were located in clinics, as fifteen additional centers were developed.

The Cuban National Program for Chronic Renal Disease, Dialysis, and Renal Transplantation occupies a singular role in Latin America, serving as an exemplary model of a program in a country with severely limited resources, yet one that provides universal health care that includes costly tertiary care for ESRD. One can only marvel at the remarkable commitment by the Cuban government to provide life-saving dialysis treatment to its citizens with kidney failure. As we shall see from the program's emphasis—not just on the provision of dialysis and transplanta-tion, but also the incorporation of systemwide efforts at prevention—the program is unique in the world (Frank, 2005; Herrera, personal com-munication, December 2006).

Health-System Organization—Chronic Renal Disease Program

As with all general and specialty care and associated research and train-ing, the Cuban Ministry of Public Health leads and directs the allocation of economic and manpower resources to the program. The specialty institutes are largely responsible for the ongoing operations of their indi-vidual programs and services, which are exercised through their leader-ship and management functions within the ministry itself (Herrera, per-sonal communication, December 2006).

At the center of the chronic renal disease program is the National Insti-tute of Nephrology in Havana, which was founded in 1966 as one of eight clinical institutes in the health system. Currently staffed by more than a hundred professionals, with specialists in thirteen fields, it directs the national renal disease program and integrates with primary-care physi-cians, specialists, clinics, and hospitals across the country. It oversees organ procurement and the national organ bank with its registry; trains specialists; and carries out about forty transplants in the institute's hospi-tal section annually—and has performed more than a thousand trans-plants since 1970. More than a hundred patients receive routine dialysis care at the institute and are often voluntary participants in ongoing clini-cal research. In addition to these inpatient and outpatient services and an intensive care unit, the institute also houses clinical labs in renal pathophysiology, transplant immunology, clinical biochemistry, nuclear medicine, preventive epidemiology, and pathology, among others.

Drs. Raúl Herrera and Miguel Almaguer, two of Cuba's leading nephrologists, based at the institute, provide visionary leadership in guiding both the clinical research directions and the development of the country's clinical renal services. Presently, the institute is responsible for forty-seven dialysis facilities, nine transplant centers, thirty-three hos-pitals for organ procurement, and five tissue-typing laboratories. Her-rera and Almaguer and their colleagues conduct research and publish widely within the regional and international specialist journals and organizations. All clinical practice and relevant research data are con-tained within a highly sophisticated database system communicating via fiber-optic connections to all dialysis facilities and transplant cen-ters in the system. This state-of-the-art system facilitates regional and/or local centers in the conduct of their own clinical evaluations, research, and quality-assurance procedures.

Despite these sophisticated technical accomplishments, entering a Cuban dialysis facility can feel like a time warp. At the bedside are machines from the last and sometimes an even earlier generation, with the effect compounded by the age and condition of some of the buildings. The experience is not dissimilar from that of seeing 1950s vintage American cars on the streets in Havana. Ironically, both are results of the long-standing U.S. embargo. Yet, despite these cosmetic differences, Cubans provide ESRD patient management that is in most other ways comparable to that in the United States.

The Cuban ESRD Program

As a direct consequence of the embargo, hemodialysis is the only available treatment modality for ESRD patients, as the solutions and disposable equipment necessary for chronic peritoneal dialysis are too costly. Typical treatment regimens, identical to those in the United States and Europe, are thrice weekly for four to five hours at maximum obtainable blood-flow rates to optimize treatment efficiency. Every patient uses disposable artificial kidneys that are of the latest generation, but all patients must reuse these kidneys because of their high cost in Cuba—another impact of the embargo. In contrast, reuse of disposables in the United States is declining, as the cost of artificial kidneys has fallen dramatically and the problems with sterilants required in the post-treatment cleaning and sterilization process have increased. As in all modern dialysis units around the globe, reverse osmosis water treatment is utilized in all Cuban facilities to remove any infectious organisms or chemical impurities from the water (Chronic kidney disease, 2006; Herrera, personal communication, December 2006).

Most treatment facilities are in regional hospitals or nearby clinics, and while the facilities are hygienic and well staffed, the buildings themselves run the gamut from modern to colonial. Despite some aesthetic shortcomings that are being steadily addressed, each facility has separate treatment areas for isolating patients infected with hepatitis C and/or B. The dialysis treatment is performed by Cuban trained and certified nurses and technicians, and, in contrast to the United States, a physician is always present within the facility, regardless of day or time. Staff must be licensed for practice, and nursing staff are university graduates with special training in nephrology. Social workers are present in the dialysis units as well. Nephrology services are accredited within Cuba as part of the general hospital accreditation process, which includes a rigorous annual on-site inspection. Linked by the information system based at the nephrology institute in Havana, reports are sent daily to the national center and local hospital directors, with baseline data, incidents, and so forth. This database permits detailed analysis of all aspects of the national program as well as individual facility operations and outcomes.

Patients have ready access to social and dietary services in each facility, and in many instances the government provides additional food allocations to assist with special nutritional needs. In certain rural areas, the government also provides temporary housing for patients who live long distances from the centers. Routine medications are subsidized by the government, and patients have access to many, but not all, newer drugs for hypertension. Chronic anemia, an ongoing and disabling aspect of kidney failure, historically often required frequent blood transfusions. In the 1980s, U.S. biotech companies pioneered a recombinant form of the kidney-produced hormone that increases red blood cell counts (erythropoietin) to counter that disabling side effect. Because the embargo prevented importation of the U.S.-manufactured drug, Cuban scientists were prompted to develop their own distinct recombinant form of the hormone, which is administered to all who require it (Fajardo, personal communication, December 2006).

Cuba has approximately 2,400 patients on dialysis at forty-six centers cared for by 425 trained specialists (includes residents in training) (Herrera, personal communication, December 2006). At less than six patients per physician, this is a remarkable ratio compared to that in the United States, where physicians may have more than ten times that number of patients in their practice (Table 8.1). Most of the dialysis facilities include physician offices, exam rooms, and specially equipped treatment rooms, which facilitates frequent examinations and reduces travel times for staff and patients, as well as hospital emergency visits.

The causes of renal failure in this population are similar to the underlying causes of hypertension, diabetes, and glomerulopathy, exactly as seen in the United States (US Renal Data System, 2007), and the Cuban ESRD incidence of 95–100 per million population (Herrera, personal communication, February 2007) is notable. These rates are below U.S. figures but substantially higher than those for the other Caribbean or

Table 8.1   Cuban ESRD Program Data 2007

Dialysis services in Cuba	47
Total patients on dialysis	2400
Total dialysis machines	447
Dialysis mortality	28.3%
Transplants-cadaver	150
Transplants-related donor	15

Source: Dr. J. F. Pérez-Oliva Diaz. Vice Director National Renal Disease Program

Latin American countries, which is understandable since, compared to Cuba, these countries offer very limited or no treatment for ESRD. However, for a program begun in the sixties, it is not entirely clear why these rates lag behind those of the United States or especially Puerto Rico, where the ethnic differences between countries are small (Chronic kidney disease, 2006). The nephrologists confirm that all patients requiring treatment are accepted into the program, but at the same time they acknowledge that prior to the 2002 expansion of facilities, some patients were not referred for care because they lived in distant rural areas without convenient access to treatment.

While the Cuban government has not released definitive, sequential morbidity and mortality data, there are statistics on treatment for more than fifteen years that speak to the overall quality of patient management. The most recent data report a 28.3 percent mortality rate in 2007, which is comparable to that of many facilities in the United States (US Renal Data System, 2007).

There are nine transplant centers, which are located in regional hospitals and the institute in Havana. Tissue typing is performed in five of them, and thirty-three hospitals participate in the organ-procurement program. The annual transplant rate for the country varies from between sixteen to twenty-two per million population per year and historically was influenced by severe fluctuations in the economy. Cadaveric sources make up 90 percent of donors, as Cuba does not transplant kidneys from living, nonrelated donors (Herrera, personal communication, February 2007).

A careful reader might be wondering about the economics of this government program. Along with the above-noted dearth of outcome statistics, cost figures are also limited. The staff at the nephrology institute notes that the average ESRD patient in Cuba costs the system around $12,000 to $15,000 (USD) per year (Herrera, personal communication, February 2007). In 2006 in the United States, Medicare alone (the program pays for all ESRD care after an initial stabilization period) paid nearly $70,000 (USD) per patient annually, and this amount does not incorporate the costs of stabilization paid by other plans (US Renal Data System, 2007).

Nephrology Integration into the Cuban Health System and the Focus on Prevention

An important outcome of the research efforts at the nephrology institute was the development of the Cuban National Program for Chronic Renal Disease, Dialysis, and Renal Transplantation, a multitiered effort that is fully integrated into the national Cuban health system. Integrating with the health system would seem to have been straightforward for the renal program in that the nephrologists had also shifted from the old paradigm of problem-oriented care to a prevention orientation that focused on the specific disease trajectory of each individual. By directing health-system efforts at prevention, early detection, and management of diseases that can lead to kidney failure, and especially at aggressive management of diabetes, the entire health system is deployed to address the humanitarian and economic impacts of the explosion of kidney failure underway not only in Cuba, but worldwide (Chronic kidney disease, 2006). Kidney failure secondary to obesity and all the associated complications related to diabetes has proved difficult to manage under any treatment regimen, and treatment of this burgeoning population is expected to cost upwards of a trillion dollars worldwide. Most nations are ill prepared for the challenge; however Cuba is addressing this problem through an integrated effort of early detection and individualized treatment that is embedded in its community-based health system (López, 2005; Working together for health, 2006).

Facing this potential for exponential growth in demand for dialysis and transplant, Cuba's leading nephrologists, Drs. Raúl Herrera and Miguel Almaguer are pioneering a research initiative through the National Institute of Nephrology in Havana that is examining the problem at the root cause. To introduce targeted preventive and treatment measures into existing health-system programs, pilot screening programs of entire resident populations have begun in two provinces and Havana. In 2005, initial findings from the Isle of Youth (80,000 population) study were published revealing heretofore unsuspected individuals with early markers indicating a propensity for the disease (Almaguer & Herrera, 2005).

In order to institute appropriate treatment and preventive measures, researchers are identifying individuals with early markers of chronic disease prior to the development of symptoms that accompany more advanced organ-system deterioration. With simple screening tests, investigators have identified far larger numbers of at-risk individuals than anticipated. Evidence is sought for cardiovascular or kidney involvement and the ubiquitous silent killer, hypertension, each of which can be managed preventively. Affected individuals are seen by an appropriate specialist to determine the cause of abnormalities found on screening. Once studies are complete, the individual is returned to the care of the local family physician. As testimony to the level of system integration, most of these doctors have undergone forty hours of specialized training in the care of patients with early and moderate renal failure, so they are well prepared to assume primary care.

The individual tracking and data-collection efforts are supported by the previously described information system; records are uploaded, and all patient-specific information is available for retrieval at the clinic site or at the nephrology institute for ongoing care and further research analysis. See Figure 8.1 below adapted from Miguel Almaguer López (American Association for World Health, 1997).

This screening program is the first of its kind in the world to examine an entire population on a near-simultaneous basis, and its importance cannot be overstated. The social and economic implications for Cuba and for the world are only beginning to be recognized as the early results, which have been favorable, begin to be fully understood. The full implications require long-term expansion of the study in Cuba and the development of similar studies throughout both the developed and developing world. Most importantly, these studies allow for early intervention in the management of hypertension, cardiovascular disease, and kidney disease with the very real potential for patient-life improvement and considerable economic benefit to the system.

Ironically, it is difficult to envision similar studies in the United States, because individuals identified as at risk would likely face the loss or denial of health insurance by many U.S. insurance companies. Cuban efforts at prevention of disease progression will likely prove even more effective when the embargo is lifted, as the U.S. blockade tragically restricts the availability of the latest and most effective versions of drugs used to combat hypertension and early kidney failure.

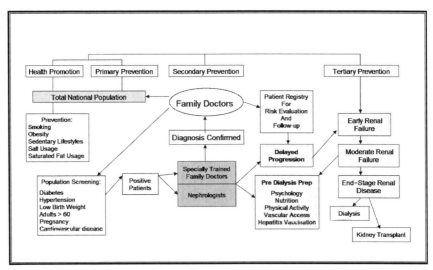

FIGURE 8.1 *Cuban National Program for the Prevention of Chronic Renal Disease*

Health Impacts of the U.S. Embargo

Cuba is the most successful among Latin American countries in providing universal health services, and especially both dialysis and transplantation to all citizens. Observers might narrowly focus on these successes and overlook the direct action of the United States that works against these humanitarian efforts—namely the U.S. embargo. For ESRD patients alone the embargo results in:

- Shortened dialysis treatments due to equipment failure and lack of backup machines;

- Shortened dialysis from increased patient load and equipment shortages;

- Chronic peritoneal dialysis not available as equipment or supplies are not obtainable;

- Only earlier-generation, used equipment is available; it must be refurbished and is often unreliable, and spare parts are nearly impossible to obtain;

- Artificial kidneys cost over $20 each (about $7 in the U.S.), as they must be purchased from distant sources;

- Mandatory reuse of disposable artificial kidneys is required owing to cost and limited availability of imported kidneys, which can reduce treatment efficiency;

- Constant shortage of disposables (IV tubing sets, blood lines, etc.) adds risk and frustration; and

- Many patent-protected pharmaceuticals are blocked, especially antihypertensive agents. (American Association for World Health, 1997)

In every scientific endeavor in Cuba, health-related or otherwise, the embargo prevents the acquisition of needed materials and equipment. The embargo renders many pieces of equipment useless without available replacement parts. Any equipment that contains 10 percent or more U.S. components requires a license from the U.S. Treasury Department, which is seldom applied for, much less approved, because the steps are deemed too arduous by U.S. companies. The ban on subsidiary trade prevents importation of necessary drugs, materials, and so on from third-country sources. International mergers and buyouts further impact those sources. Cuban shipping costs exceed those of other countries, since ships are banned from U.S. ports for 180 days after delivering cargo to Cuba.

Summary

Lying within a region that has national poverty rates of greater than 40 percent and health-care systems to match, Cuba, though also resource poor, is both a regional model and a world model with its constitutionally mandated, universal health-care system. Cuba has taken free, universal health care to levels unimaginable to the Western mind with its inclusion of kidney dialysis and transplantation among the services provided, as they are among the most costly forms of life-saving treatment in most countries.

In order to provide comprehensive care within strict cost structures, the Cuban health-care system dumped the prevailing curative model, shifting to a directed emphasis on prevention. This focus within the kidney program supported the development of a population-screening program that is, on its own, a world-class model for early detection, analysis, and treatment. Integration of the kidney program, both operationally and technologically, facilitates the long-term management of individuals identified by screening tests.

Working against the constraints of the U.S. embargo, which severely impacts availability of equipment and disposables, Cuba provides dialysis to all renal-failure patients in forty-seven centers around the country and transplantation in nine, with outcomes that exceed those of other resource-poor countries and match those of many U.S. centers.

Clearly, the Cuban health system provides a dynamic, world-class model that developing and developed countries alike should seek to understand in more detail. It offers a viable, functional approach to the provision of comprehensive health care by its effective and powerful demonstration that the provision of universal health care is not necessarily as dependent on a country's economic status as on the mustering of political will.

References

Almaguer, M., & Herrer, R. (2005). Primary health care strategies for the prevention of end-stage renal disease in Cuba. *Kidney International, 68*, Supplement 97, S4–S10.

Chronic kidney disease in the developing world: An iceberg turned into a volcano. (2006). Editorial in *MEDICC Review, VII*(5), 1–2.

Denial of food and medicine: The impact of the U.S. embargo on health and nutrition in Cuba. (1997). American Association for World Health.

Frank, M. (2005). Roundtable with two generations of Cuban nephrologists. *MEDICC Review, VII*(5), 10–12.

Herrera, R. (2005). Cuba's national program for chronic kidney disease, dialysis and transplantation, *MEDICC Review, VII*(5), 2–5.

López, M. (2005). Effect of primary health care on prevention of chronic kidney disease in Cuba. *MEDICC Review, VII*(5), 14–16.

US Renal Data System. (2007).

Working together for health. (2006). *The World Health Report.* World Health Organization.

Glossary

Acute renal failure (ARF): A time-limited form of kidney failure in which the kidney recovers function, but the individual requires temporary use of dialysis, either peritoneal or hemodialysis.

Artificial kidney: Also called a *dialyzer,* a membrane-containing device that separates the blood from the cleansing solution. Most common are bundles of synthetic hollow fibers in which the blood flows through the fiber and the solution around the outside.

Artificial kidney machine: Also called a dialysis machine and often used (confusingly) interchangeably with artificial kidney. It mixes the solution that flows on the opposite of the membrane as the blood and controls the temperature and flow rate of blood.

Chronic renal failure: Used to describe individuals with compromised renal function from a variety of causes. Tends to be progressive, though not always, and pace of deterioration varies widely from months to years and can be treated with medications and diet to slow onset of the symptoms of end-stage renal disease.

Dialysis: Used to describe the process by which an individual's system is cleansed of the buildup of impurities as a result of renal failure. It has two forms: hemodialysis and peritoneal dialysis.

End-stage renal disease (ESRD): A level of renal function that requires some form of dialysis or transplantation for survival. Symptoms of chronic renal failure become prominent at less than 15 percent of normal function.

Hemodialysis: Can be used in acute cases and in end-stage renal disease (ESRD). An external circuit of blood is pumped through an artificial kidney (a dialyzer) in which a synthetic membrane permits the transfer of impurities from the bloodstream into a fluid pumped in opposite direction on the other side of the membrane.

Peritoneal Dialysis: Can be used in acute or chronic renal failure and is accomplished by flushing the abdominal cavity with fluids through a temporary or permanent catheter (tubing). Fluid cycling allows the impurities to transfer across abdominal membranes.

CHAPTER NINE

HIV/AIDS in Cuba

Susan E. Mason

".. . protection of your partner against HIV and STI's in general is a sign of caring, and that means it's a responsibility of both partners in a relationship."

—Mariela Castro,
Director of Cuba's National Center for Sex Education

The AIDS epidemic continues worldwide. There are currently thirty-three million people living with HIV/AIDS, with 2.7 million infected in 2007. Nevertheless, the number of newly infected people is declining (UNAIDS, 2008). This, unfortunately, may not be the case in Cuba, where the incidence of the infection is rising even as the HIV infection rate is the lowest in the Americas (just 0.1 percent) and among the lowest in the world. The number of people living with HIV in Cuba has risen from approximately 2,400 in 2001 to 6,200 in 2007 (UNAIDS, 2008). According to experts within Cuba, the greatest increase has been among men having sex with men (Pérez et al., 2004). One possible explanation for this increase is a national effort to test large numbers of people in the population, especially those who may present the greatest risks, such as homosexual men. This leads to a lower number of unidentified HIV infections and a higher number of identified persons with HIV. In many countries it is common for large numbers of people to be unaware of their infection. For example, in the United States it is estimated that there are from 252,000 to 312,000 people with unidentified HIV (CDC, 2006). In Cuba, as in many countries, the stigma associated with having HIV/AIDS presents a challenge to health providers in identifying and treating people who would benefit from treatment. Nevertheless, health activists along with the staff of the Cuban Ministry of Public Health (MINSAP) continue to work at prevention, identification, and treatment. This chapter reviews the effort to manage HIV/AIDS within the context of Cuban culture and the country's emphasis on community health care. Although most information is taken from the latest reports of the status of HIV/AIDS programs in Cuba, the author includes observations from visits to key sites where HIV infection is addressed.

Prevention

In Cuba, as elsewhere, prevention makes economic sense in that it costs less to promote behavioral changes than to treat HIV/AIDS. Cuban health officials regularly use disease prevention as a way to rally the community in support of the government's efforts to keep Cubans healthy. Maintaining good health is a citizen's duty according to Cuban revolutionary ideology, and promoting good health can be viewed as an integral part of the Cuban national identity (Johnson, 2006; Schwab, 1999).

Prevention efforts focus on two vulnerable groups, males having sex with males and women who may be their partners. Cuban statistics show that the group with the highest incidence rate of HIV/AIDS today is males having sex with males (de Arazoza et al., 2007; Pérez et al., 2004). The tourist industry that brings needed hard currency to the island also brings men seeking homosexual partners and the possibility of spreading HIV. Although the sex trade involving both genders is illegal, economic incentives keep it thriving. Tourists may pay for sex with hard currency, but today they more commonly offer material goods such as clothing, sneakers, and high-status watches. In interviews with male sex workers, Hodge (2003) found these methods of payment from male tourists to be prevalent.

In response to the risks that tourist sex brings to the island, prevention programs targeting vulnerable groups and young people have permeated schools, hospitals, and even prisons. In 1998, the National Center for HIV/AIDS and STD Prevention opened with the goal of getting community members involved in the public-health effort to prevent the spread of HIV infection. Community-based physicians and health workers, school personnel, and groups including the Committee for the Defense of the Revolution and the Federation of Cuban Women work together to alert people to the dangers of HIV infection and the methods of prevention. People living with HIV/AIDS are encouraged to join prevention projects by giving talks at schools and public meetings, manning telephone hotlines, and working at testing facilities. The prevention campaign that focuses on stopping the spread of the virus encourages HIV/AIDS patients to continue taking medications, and it educates them about how to keep the virus from spreading. Specially trained counselors go into the communities to lend support to people who have HIV/AIDS and to their families. With a housing shortage in Havana, people living with HIV/AIDS are likely to remain in apartments or houses with immediate and often extended families. This means that family members require education and support from the counselors (Gorry, 2008; Pérez et al., 2004).

Attitudes about the Use of Condoms as a Method of Prevention

Cuban resistance to the use of condoms was cited in an article in the *Lancet* medical journal as far back as 1997, and it appears that it may persist today. At a conference at Cuba's internationally known Pedro Kouri Institute of Tropical Medicine, the message delivered was that Cubans generally do not like to use condoms with other Cubans (Burr, 1997). Whether they use them in relations with foreign tourists is questionable, and from the increase in HIV/AIDS incidence rates, the answer may be in the negative.

The government's response to condom resistance has been to distribute quality condoms either free of charge or for very small amounts of money. Condoms are sold very inexpensively in restaurants, cafeterias, bars, and pharmacies. Special projects have included free condom distribution and education in health clinics, beauty salons, and by young people on rollerblades giving them away on the streets of Havana (Gorry, 2008).

In addition to condom distribution, the work of the National Center for Sex Education (CENESEX) has focused on changing a culture that has been resistant to safe-sex practices. Directed by Mariela Castro, Raúl Castro's daughter and Fidel's niece, CENESEX has focused on behavioral changes that are tied to the culture of "macho." According to an interview published in *MEDICC Review* in 2006, Mariela Castro stated that the mission of CENESEX is to contribute to "the development of a culture of sexuality that is full, pleasurable and responsible, as well as to promote the full exercise of sexual rights" (Reed, 2006, p. 8). When speaking about HIV, she emphasizes the word "responsible," especially as it relates to using condoms. She distinguishes between macho and manly, the former involving the use of sex as power over women and the latter engaging in "equitable, respectful relationships" (Reed, 2006,

p. 8). She points out that simply telling men to use condoms is not likely to be effective; a better approach is to change attitudes about what it means to be a man, that responsible behavior is masculine and loving, not only for a man's partners but also for his own health. The work of CENESEX is to educate through programs in schools, the media, posters, and television.

A talk by Mariela Castro at CENESEX communicated essentially the same message, that although there have been great strides in promoting the idea that protection means prevention—and more importantly that protection means love—there is more to be done. In listening to Castro and her colleagues at CENESEX, it is clear that they are passionate and persistent in pursuing their goals of promoting sexual rights and responsibilities. The plight of married women who contract HIV from their husbands was addressed as a national problem. Mariela Castro openly asserted that when men do not use condoms they may be endangering their wives and potentially their children. She also discussed the stigma attached to people who are openly homosexual, transsexual, or engage in transvestite behavior. Largely through her efforts, Cuba provides sex-change operations on request. It is unquestionable that Mariela Castro's position and personal influence has advanced the cause of sexual responsibility in Cuba, but when asked about her role in influencing change, she responded that there was still much to be accomplished.

Figure 9.1 shows how HIV/AIDS prevention programs are organized to target vulnerable groups in the community.

FIGURE 9.1 *National Program of Prevention HIV/AIDS Cuba, 2003*

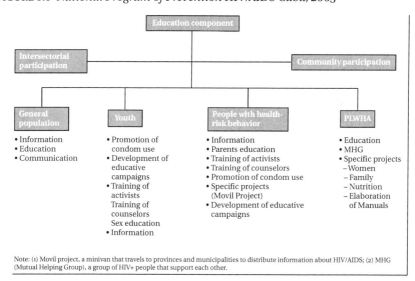

Note: (1) Movil project, a minivan that travels to provinces and municipalities to distribute information about HIV/AIDS; (2) MHG (Mutual Helping Group), a group of HIV+ people that support each other.

Pérez et al., p. 11.

The Hidden Side of the Moon

The Hidden Side of the Moon, a popular soap opera first shown on Cuban television in 2006, presents characters that discuss HIV, AIDS, and homosexuality. In one episode, a young teenage girl contracts the virus, and in another, a young woman discovers that her husband is having sex with men. While the show brought about a great deal of controversy and disagreement among Cubans, it was very popular. The decision to put it on prime-time TV resulted from what a Cuban television official called the continuing of high-risk behavior that spreads HIV/AIDS (Matos, 2006). CENESEX helped produce the series.

The soap opera episodes showing the wife learning of her husband's sexual infidelities with men represents a serious subject in a country where most women contract HIV/AIDS from their husbands and most men get it from sex with other men. Interviews conducted with HIV-positive women between 2000 and 2005 revealed that 70.9 percent had husbands who were having sex with men (de Arazoza et al., 2007). The same study found that in 2005 men having sex with men resulted in 85.3 percent of the HIV-positive cases. By bringing bisexual activity to prime-time television along with a discussion about HIV, the goal was to get people to openly discuss the spread of AIDS and its prevention.

Identifying HIV/AIDS in Cuba

The process of identifying people who are HIV-positive or have symptoms of AIDS takes place in the community, in the schools, hospitals, community centers, workplaces, and prisons. Community-based doctors test on a voluntary basis people in high-risk groups: men having sex with men, women married to these men, teenagers who are known to have multiple sex partners, and pregnant women. Testing is mandatory for prison inmates, persons entering the military, and persons traveling abroad. If a person is confirmed as HIV-positive, he or she must provide a list of past and current sexual contacts, all of whom are tested on a voluntary basis. Anyone who wishes to be tested but does not fit into one of these categories can go to one of many anonymous testing sites (Gorry, 2008; Johnson, 2006; Pérez et al., 2004). The total number of tests performed each year was estimated in 2004 to be between 1.5 and 1.6 million (Pérez et al., 2004). There is little vertical transmission, that is, from mother to baby, because women who are HIV-positive are placed on medication to suppress the virus or are encouraged to abort. If they do choose to have the baby, Cesarean sections are performed to lessen the rate of transmission, and they refrain from breastfeeding, which also reduces the risk (Castro, Khawja, & González-Nuñez, 2007). When someone is diagnosed with the virus, careful monitoring takes place either in state-run sanatoria or by medical professionals in the community.

The strategy for identification of all infectious diseases in Cuba is outlined by Cooper, Kennelly, and Orduñez-García (2006) in their discussion of the Cuban health system. Once there is an effective vaccine, the goal is to immunize the entire population beginning with the most vulnerable groups. When a vaccine is not available, there is screening of the people most likely to contract the disease. The community is mobilized to screen and treat, so that local involvement becomes key in finding the people who need to be treated. Children are given special attention and are monitored from the pre-conception to the well-baby phase, thereby reducing infant mortality and helping to produce healthy children.

Using this strategy and the combined efforts of the National Center for HIV/AIDS and STD Prevention, CENESEX, the Federation of Cuban Women, the Committee for the Defense of the Revolution, schools, and community health providers, Cuba has managed to maintain at 0.1 percent the lowest HIV rate among Caribbean nations. Even with an increase in incidence, Cuba's efforts at preventing and identifying HIV seem to be paying off. Once the virus is detected in an individual, the treatment begins. It is mandatory and without cost to the patient and family.

Treatment: Community versus Sanatoria

Today, treatment of HIV/AIDS for most Cubans takes place in the community. From 2001, the country's pharmaceutical industry has produced eight antiretroviral drugs for the treatment of AIDS, resulting in a decline in deaths and related opportunistic infections (Castro et al., 2008). Prior to 1993, people with HIV/AIDS were required to live quarantined in one of fourteen sanatoria. These sanatoria resembled suburban communities, with private apartments, gardens, and health-care facilities on site. Residents were given high-quality food and medicine at no charge and were free to socialize with other residents. According to a study by Castro and colleagues (Castro et al., 2008), women with HIV infection often became pregnant at the sanatoria because there were no restrictions on unprotected sex, and, at that time, physicians were unaware that re-infection with different strains of the virus could occur. In most cases, the women aborted, but some did carry to term with mixed transmission results. Today, more HIV-positive women are deciding to have babies, and the antiretroviral therapy program (ART) in Cuba has made this possible.

The sanatoria that were mandatory between 1986 and 1993 brought considerable international controversy. AIDS activists charged that they were essentially prisons, and that it was unethical to force people with HIV infection to leave their homes and families because of their illness (Fink, 2003). In defense, Cuban officials and some scholars who studied the sanatoria firsthand stated that the treatment of people with HIV/AIDS was consistent with treatment of Cubans with other infectious diseases and that no Cuban or international law was broken (Chomsky, 2000; Farmer, 2003). Nevertheless, by 1993, although the sanatoria remained open, they were no longer mandatory except for people unable or unwilling to comply with treatment in the community (Gorry, 2008). Most people living with AIDS (PLWA) today are treated in the community, but some choose to live in the sanatoria for short amounts of time because of its advantages. Residents in the three-to-six-month sanatoria programs receive high-quality food, medication, close monitoring of symptoms, psychological evaluations, and their full work salary. In 2003, 40 percent of people with HIV/AIDS had spent some voluntary time in Cuba's sanatoria (Pérez et al., 2004).

In 1997, AZT was introduced into Cuba and in 2001 antiretroviral drugs (ART) became available. These medications allowed people to be treated successfully in their own communities by their neighborhood doctors. But the availability of medication was not the end of the story. People living with AIDS had to take their medication, they had to practice safe sex, and they had to live with stigma.

People first diagnosed with HIV who choose to live at home are required to attend a day clinic every day for several months before their care is turned over to their family doctor. During this initial time period, they are carefully assessed, monitored, and provided with extra food to build up their defenses. They are registered with a central agency that provides them with antiretroviral medications (ART) produced in Cuba. They attend education sessions where they are taught about the expected progression of the virus, safe-sex practices, and their rights (Pérez et al., 2004).

Compliance to medication regimens and safe-sex practices are encouraged through regular meetings held in communities where people with HIV/AIDS support each other, learn about new protocols, and discuss their rights. Patients are asked to volunteer to help others to comply with treatment, to talk to young people in schools, and to become AIDS activists for the benefit of their communities. When patients do not comply, they are visited in their homes by nurses who work with families to achieve compliance through education and medication-management plans. For all people living with HIV/AIDS in the community, medication compliance is monitored by tests conducted by physicians and nurses (Pérez et al., 2004). Compliance is mandatory, and when patients cannot manage in the community, they are sent to a sanatoria (Gorry, 2008).

Stigma Associated with HIV/AIDS

Stigma for people living with AIDS exists in Cuba as in most countries, including the United States (Brown, Trujillo, & Macintyre, 2001). To assist in reducing stigma and unfair treatment, health-care workers are required to take a twenty-hour course on treating people with dignity (Gorry, 2008). In Cuba, the largest number of new cases are men having sex with men, and for many Cuban men who are homosexual there remains substantial discrimination. Anti-gay attitudes continue to be pervasive throughout the island (Johnson, 2006; Voss, 2008). Government campaigns that support sexual diversity are ongoing today through education and media productions, with the goals of reducing stigma and encouraging people to get tested for HIV and to get support if tested positive (Gorry, 2008). Although homosexuality is legal, police are still known to harass individuals who display openly gay behaviors. This level of stigma, coupled with having HIV/AIDS, results in a substantial burden on individuals who are homosexual and infected and also on health-care providers who are required to identify, assess, and treat them in the community.

Women living with HIV/AIDS who are pregnant or wish to have a child are another group that faces substantial stigma. The vertical transmission rate, from mother to child, is extremely low, with estimates as low as twenty-nine known cases since 1986. The actual number is likely to be higher, but, nevertheless, transmission rates are reduced through programs that offer abortions during the first twelve weeks of pregnancy, antiretroviral medications without charge, Cesarean births, and baby formula instead of breast milk (Castro et al., 2008; de Arazoza et al., 2007). Increasingly, women are choosing to forgo abortions and are carrying to term. In a study of fifty-five women with HIV infection, it was reported that many felt discrimination by members of their community. Several women stated that having a child who was free of the virus helped people to accept them but that having HIV still carry substantial stigma (Castro et al., 2008).

Where is Cuba Today with HIV/AIDS?

Cuba is meeting the challenge of the effects of globalization on the infection incidence of HIV/AIDS. Cuba's strict antidrug policy and enforcement has resulted in well over 99 percent (Castro et al., 2007) of HIV infections being transmitted through sexual relations. The Cuban response has been to test large segments of the population, about 1.5 million people each year (Pérez et al., 2004), and to mandate treatment of all identified HIV-infected people quickly and without charge. Most treatment is in the community with structured programs aimed at preventing further spread. This strategy has resulted in a 0.1 percent (UNAIDS, 2008) prevalence rate and a likely low number of unidentified cases. Cuba produces its own antiretroviral medications at a capacity that is striving to keep up with its present and future needs (Gorry, 2008). For a country of eleven million people with an economy that has suffered from economic downturns and the U.S.-initiated embargo, this is quite an achievement.

References

Brown, L., Trujillo, L., & Macintyre, K. (2001). Interventions to reduce HIV/AIDS stigma: What have we learned? The Population Council/Horizons Program, New Orleans: Tulane School of Public Health and Tropical Medicine. Retrieved on October 21, 2008, from, www.popcouncil.org/pdfs/horizons/litrvwstigdisc.pdf

Burr, C. (1997, Aug. 30). Assessing Cuba's approach to contain AIDS and HIV. *Lancet, 350,* 647.

Castro, A., Khawja, Y., & González-Nuñez, I. (2007). Sexuality, reproduction, and HIV in women: The impact of antiretroviral therapy in elective pregnancies in Cuba. *AIDS, 21*(suppl. 5), S49–S54.

Castro, A., Khawja, Y., & González-Nuñez, I. (2008, July–August). Giving birth, contesting stigma: Cuban women living with HIV. *NACLA Report on the Americas. A Cautious Hope, HIV/AIDS in Latin America, 41*(4), 25–29. New York: North American Congress on Latin America.

CDC (2006, June 2). MMWR Weekly. *Epidemiology of HIV/AIDS—United States, 1981–2005.* Retrieved on September 29, 2008, from, http://www.cdc.gov/mmwr/preview/mmwrhtml/mm5521a2.htm

Chomsky, A. (2000). The threat of a good example: Health and revolution in Cuba. In J. Y. Kim, J. V. Mullen, A. Irwin, & J. Gershman (Eds.), *Dying for growth: Global inequality and the health of the poor* (pp. 331–357). Monroe, ME: Common Courage Press.

Cooper, R. S., Kennelly, J. F., & Orduñez-García, P. (2006). Health in Cuba. *International Journal of Epidemiology, 35*(4), 817–824.

de Arazoza, H., Joanes, J., Lounes, R., Legeai, C., Clemencon, S., Pérez, J., et al. (2007). The HIV/AIDS epidemic in Cuba: Description and tentative explanation of its low HIV prevalence. *Biomedical Central (BMC) Infectious Diseases, 7*(130). Retrieved on November 18, 2008, from http://www.biomedcentral.com/1471-2334/7/130

Farmer, P. (2003). *Pathologies of power, human rights and the new war of the poor.* Berkeley, CA: University of California Press.

Fink, S. (2003). Cuba's energetic AIDS doctor. *American Journal of Public Health, 93*(5), 712–716.

Gorry, C. (Fall, 2008). Cuba's HIV/AIDS program: Controversy, care and cultural shift. *MEDDIC Review, 10*(4), 10–14.

Hodge, G. D. (2003). Colonizing the Cuban body. In A. Chomsky, B. Carr, & P. M. Smorkaloff (Eds.), *The Cuba reader* (pp. 628–634). Durham, NC: Duke University Press.

Johnson, C. (2006). Health as culture and nationalism in Cuba. *Canadian Journal of Latin American and Caribbean Studies, 31*(61), 91–113.

Matos, O. (2006, April 20). Cuba: Not everyone's ready for AIDS story on prime time TV. *The Amsterdam News*, p. 2.

Pérez, J., Pérez, D., Gonzalez, I., Diaz Jidy, M., Orta, M., Aragones, C., et al. (2004). Approaches to the management of HIV/AIDS in Cuba: A case study. Geneva: World Health Organization. Retrieved on September 28, 2008, from http://www.who.int/hiv/amds/case1.pdf

Reed, G. A. (March/April, 2006). MR interview: Mariela Castro, MS, director, National Center for Sex Education. *MEDICC Review, 8*(1), 8–9. Retrieved on 03/11/09 at http://www.medicc.org/publications/medicc_review/pdf-files/0406.pdf

Report on the global AIDS epidemic. (2008). Retrieved on November 18, 2008, from http://www.unaids.org/en/KnowlegeCentre/HIVData/GlobalReport/2008/2008_Global_report.asp

Schwab, P. (1999). *Cuba: Confronting the U.S. embargo.* New York: St. Martin's Press.

Voss, M. (2008, March 27). Castro champions gay rights in Cuba. BBC News. Retrieved on October 9, 2008, from http://news.bbc.co.uk/2/hi/americas/7314845.stm

CHAPTER TEN

Beyond Health Services: Channeling Capacity to Manage Health Determinants

Jerry Spiegel

Discussion of Cuba's remarkable health achievements has especially highlighted the role of health services (de la Torre, Márquez, Gutiérrez Muñiz, López Pardo, & Rojas Ochoa, 2004; Feinsilver, 1993; Field, 2006; MacDonald, 1999; Whiteford & Branch, 2008). This is understandable, as there is indeed much to marvel at in the manner in which health care has been made universally accessible and delivered with considerable innovation amid the country's resource constraints. Nonetheless, this only tells part of the story.

Amid the growing worldwide disparities that have accompanied increased globalization from the latter part of the twentieth century onward, we have come to more comprehensively appreciate that health consequences are attributable to a wide range of influences. The World Health Organization's (WHO) Commission on Social Determinants of Health (CSDH) concluded that "at the global level, we now understand, better than at any moment in history, how social factors affect health and health equity" (CSDH, 2007, p. 34). These observations were then reinforced by the commission's final report in 2008.

This chapter examines how efforts to meet the health needs of Cubans have included systematic processes targeting the determinants of health to promote equity. It reflects on the basic policy underpinnings for this, especially how concepts such as "intersectorality" and "community capacity" have been central to such implementation. It then presents three distinct case-study scenarios in which this can be observed: tackling extremely difficult economic circumstances during the "special period"; addressing the threat of acute health crisis caused by outbreaks of dengue fever; and meeting the challenges of growth through tourism expansion. Why and how these efforts were able to be undertaken, and undertaken successfully, and factors such as "social capital" and "political will," considered not as rhetorical concepts but as constructs that can systematically be observed in examining how health determinants can be addressed in any society—not just in the context of the fascinating "Cuban natural experiment"—will be examined.

Putting Alma-Ata into Practice

PRIMARY HEALTH CARE

In many ways, the evolution of Cuba's health policy has closely echoed the principles for primary health care that were enunciated by the WHO's International Health Conference in Alma-Ata in 1978:

> Primary health care is essential health care based on practical, scientifically sound and socially acceptable methods and technology made universally accessible to individuals and families in the community through their full participation and at a cost that the community and country can afford to maintain at every stage of their development in the spirit of self reliance and self-determination . . ." (WHO-UNICEF, 1978, p. 1).

Although the "Declaration of Alma Ata" was endorsed by the WHO executive board and ratified by the member states of the World Health Assembly, events of the subsequent two decades such as the expansion of globalization and neoliberalism, weakening public-health expenditures, and privatization (Harvey, 2005) served to fundamentally undermine adherence to the ambitious call for achieving "Health for All" by the year 2000 (Maciocco et al., 2008). The Alma-Ata vision, at root, challenged many countries' prevailing power bases in three distinct ways: (1) seeking alternatives to the "medical model" as a way to achieve health; (2) calling on government to actively fulfill a central role; and (3) stressing the importance of public participation and empowerment.

From the beginning, Cuba adopted the vision extolled at Alma-Ata. The success achieved by Cuba provides strong evidence of the efficacy of the policies endorsed in 1978. It provided proof that the policies could indeed work if seriously implemented and if specific contextual factors were addressed. In many countries, the policy options promoted by institutions such as the World Bank and International Monetary Fund left little space for the basic thrust of Alma-Ata to survive, let alone thrive (Brown, Cueto, & Fee, 2006; Maciocco et al., 2008).

A "Natural Experiment"

I have argued elsewhere (Spiegel & Yassi, 2004) that Cuba's relatively unique geopolitical position "on the margins of globalization" provided distinct circumstances in that Cuba lay outside of the economic and social pressures that were rendering adherence to the Alma-Ata vision extremely difficult, a position also put forward by Whiteford and Branch (2008). In this context, although the U.S. attempts to isolate Cuba undeniably contributed much to Cuba's economic difficulties, it inadvertently also contributed to the feasibility of a "policy space" that enabled a prominent state role alongside a model that relied on strong community involvement.

Cuba's unique position was vividly described by Cuban President Fidel Castro when he provocatively suggested that Cuba was able to achieve its undeniable success in areas such as health "thanks to its privileged position as a non-member of the International Monetary Fund" (Castro Ruiz, 2002). This was more than a rhetorical jab. The reality is that Cuba was indeed independent of the structural adjustment policy pressures on low- and middle-income countries to reduce public-sector expenditures in other settings (Breman & Shelton, 2001; Labonte & Schrecker, 2007).

The Alma-Ata vision of primary health care was not at all silent with regard to "social determinants of health," and explicitly called for a broad, multisectoral effort to be undertaken, that is, one extending over and above the organization of health services:

> It [PHC] involves, in addition to the health sector, all related sectors and aspects of national and community development, in particular agriculture, animal husbandry, food, industry, education, housing, public works, communications and other sectors; and demands the coordinated efforts of all those sectors. (WHO-UNICEF, 1978, Section VII(4))

The neoliberal presumption that health is best achieved by having it "trickle down" as a result of economic growth (Dollar, 2001; Dollar & Kraay, 2002), on the other hand, provided a vision of intersectoral interaction that placed considerable faith in how the market's "invisible hand" could stimulate optimal results with limited attention to state involvement in public-health infrastructure. This positing of economic growth as the best foundation for public policy (World Bank, 1993) unashamedly discounted the need to explicitly invest in strong national and local health systems and PHC units, let alone establish fundamental institutional capacity for pursuing healthy public policy across different sectors. In fact, the value of establishing coherent, core health-service capacity at different governance levels was largely neglected and replaced by an explicit emphasis on vertically implemented selective (versus comprehensive) care strategies on the grounds that these could be more cost-effectively delivered. (Brown et al., 2006; Maciocco et al., 2008). This emphasis on groups of so-called targeted interventions was later echoed by the WHO's Commission on Macroeconomics and Health (World Health Organization, 2003), which again tended to underplay the importance of basic health-system coherence, failing even to consider this worthy as a realistic option to consider implementing. And further emphasis on "vertical" programs largely directed by external donors has further extended this orientation.

Before proceeding to case study examinations of how Cuba, in various settings, denied the neoliberal model, it is useful to first consider the institutional context constructed in Cuba to address this matter.

INTERSECTORALITY

In a workshop exploring the "intersectoral management of health" that our Canadian-Cuban team held in Havana in 2008 (Spiegel et al., 2008b), Dr. Pastor Castell of Cuba's National School of Public Health, author of the basic Cuban study on this subject (Castell, 2007), referred to intersectorality as both a "philosophy" and a "technology." By *philosophy*, he refers to the ideas laid out in the Alma-Ata declaration that have been elaborated in various writings dealing with the determinants of health. *Technology*, however, refers to the institutional practices that can be and are applied systematically to a range of different values and priorities in relation to efforts to effectively improve health.

In Cuba, the systematic organization of health services as part of a nationally integrated system provides a basic framework that comprehensively connects the people professionally involved in the enterprise of improving health.

The organization of health services in Cuba is not only well integrated with basic units staffed by well-trained people at the national, provincial, municipal, and local levels, but there is notably a "space" for health to be explicitly integrated with other sectors in health councils that exist at each level. This was especially strengthened in the early 1990s by the establishment of the people's councils as the basic level of governance and local advocacy to which delegates were elected. The establishment of the *Comisión de Calidad de Vida y Salud* [Commission on Quality of Life and Health] at the national level has further reinforced the extent of accountability and oversight that has helped to maintain the profile of health-related issues.

COMMUNITY CAPACITY

In addition to ensuring a credible health- and public-sector presence at different levels of governance from the locally elected delegates at the People's Power people's councils through to higher levels, provision is well-established for giving voice and space for citizens to systematically raise concerns (Dilla & Oxhorn, 2002; Roman, 1999). So-called mass organizations such as the Committees for the Defense of the Revolution (CDR) and the Cuban Federation of Women (FMC), which had been created by the government as early as 1960 to provide organized options for public participation, do not eliminate the need and usefulness for other ad hoc forms of organization. Rather, they provide a venue for raising issues so that both public involvement and identification of concerns are possible, as will be illustrated in the case studies below. Mass organization, building on the high level of literacy that was achieved as one of the first consolidated accomplishments of the Cuban Revolution (Macdonald, 1985), have further reinforced the foundation for empowering the systematic participation of citizens in defense of their interests.

Case Studies

CAYO HUESO: A VULNERABLE INNER-CITY COMMUNITY IN THE "SPECIAL PERIOD"

An unintended consequence of post-1959 Cuba's favoring of previously neglected rural and secondary urban areas was a deterioration of the infrastructure of the 450-year-old capital city of Havana, and especially its most vulnerable inner-city communities. For example, between 1962 and 1972, while the city contained 27 percent of the country's population, it only received 15 percent of all new housing (Coyula & Hamberg, 2003; Young, 1985).

The need to address the social, environmental, and economic problems in the capital had been strongly asserted by local community members in the mid-1980s, and planning was initiated to deal with this. In this context, the Group for the Integral Development of the Capital (GDIC) was established in 1987 by the Cuban government to strengthen local capacity for responding to Havana's deterioration (Chappotin, 1998); and in 1988 the *Talleres de Transformación Integral del Barrio*

[Integrated Neighborhood Transformation Workshops] were launched as a GDIC pilot project. The *talleres* were to mobilize local professionals to form interdisciplinary teams to work at the community level in a decentralized and participatory manner. Initially, these *talleres* focused on improving housing conditions, urban education for children and youth, community identity, and the local economy and were successful in securing funds from foreign sources to address a variety of community health concerns. The *talleres* existed alongside the various mass organizations and interacted systematically with the recently established people's councils to strengthen community participation in resolving local issues.

The so-called special period, which followed the collapse of the Socialist bloc and its trade with Cuba, had a serious and widespread impact on health, the environment, and social services in Cuba (more specifically, on nutrition, transport, water quality, housing, and public-health services) (Garfield & Santana, 1997; Kirkpatrick, 1997; Schwab, 1999). Central Havana, the most densely populated and one of the oldest of the fifteen municipalities within the City of Havana, experienced increasing rates of infectious and noncommunicable diseases as well as injuries. Infrastructure difficulties encompassed housing, access to potable water, and disposal of liquid and solid waste; while disease vectors were prevalent, and diarrhoeal diseases, leptospirosis, tuberculosis, and sexually transmitted diseases had increased (INHEM, 1999; Yassi et al., 1999).

"PLAN CAYO HUESO"

In Cayo Hueso, one of Central Havana's five people's council areas, 70 percent of the houses were classified by the Municipal Department of Housing as "bad," with 38 percent categorized as "uninhabitable." Having become aware of the needs of Cayo Hueso through the efforts of the local people's council delegates and mass organizations, the Cuban government initiated a concentrated initiative between 1995 and 1999 to improve the quality of life and human health in this neighborhood. The plan mobilized government organizations as well as nongovernmental organizations (NGOs), and was implemented as an organized set of interventions in coordination with the provincial and municipal governments. Interest in this undertaking was secured by a massive advertising campaign on radio and television as well as face-to-face meetings promoting Plan Cayo Hueso as a plan to improve living conditions, health, and well-being. In order to promote participation in collective projects, this campaign emphasized the value of volunteer work.

This mass mobilization of local and national resources targeted the repair of housing exteriors and subsidies for repairing interiors, the repair of public buildings and construction of new venues, the repair of streets and replacement of water and drainage infrastructure, improvement of solid waste removal, installation of improved lighting, and improvement of neighborhood social and cultural activities, as well as health promotion (Spiegel et al., 2001).

To coordinate the infrastructural upgrades and exterior building repairs being undertaken with the aid of the ministries and NGOs, the municipal government established the Office of Rehabilitation Development (ORD) to oversee and coordinate activities. In addition, the *taller* continued to build spaces where youth and children could gather, and, along with the CDR and FMC, continued their health-promotion programs, conducting, for example, several programs for seniors such as self-esteem workshops and exercise programs. Above all, the improvements were undertaken with and for the benefit of the affected populations, not for a gentrification plan that would prompt their marginalization and ultimate migration.

COPING WITH DIFFICULTY

So that lessons from the actions taken could inform other communities, the head of the Cayo Hueso people's council contacted Cuban environmental health specialists to conduct a participatory action research evaluation as part of the efforts undertaken. This set the stage for an international collaboration with Canadian researchers experienced in applying an ecosystem approach to human health, forming the base for an enriching partnership (Bonet et al., 2007; Spiegel, Garcia, Yassi, & Bonet, 2005; Yassi et al., 1999).

Rigorous evaluation (Spiegel et al., 2001; 2003) confirmed that greater improvements to housing, local infrastructure, and risk exposure were more consistently perceived to have occurred in Cayo Hueso than elsewhere, especially regarding benefit to the community rather than residents' own households. This was especially observed for the most vulnerable subgroups (such as elderly women and young people under age twenty) who received targeted programs (Table 10.1). Comparison with the 1996 risk-perception survey also revealed that there was a significant decrease in perceived risk from housing conditions in the community following the intervention (Tate et al., 2003). Overall, the Cayo Hueso Plan was considered highly successful in improving the quality of life amid difficult circumstances.

Participation varied by leadership role within the community (Yassi et al., 2003). For example, while the FMC and the CDR did not make decisions, they were directly involved in mobilizing the community to participate in interventions taking place. The delegates were responsible for decision making, and they coordinated the dissemination of information regarding the interventions. Informal leaders and health professionals had a very limited role, participating only when their collaboration was requested. The community leaders (such as those active in the *taller*) acted as a link between the government and the community and facilitated greater cooperation. Although community members were not included in the decision making in the allocation of resources or in the division of labor, they were able to express their concerns about how well their needs were being met. The leaders also played an extremely important role in the dissemination of information and the mobilization of the community, thus providing the community with opportunity to participate. This complemented spontaneous forms of participation, such as that by the group of women who called themselves "Marianas" and took it upon themselves to mobilize other women to help with support efforts such as cleaning and providing snacks, but also organizing activities for children and cultural events.

It is important to note that provision of food was a significant contribution given the crisis conditions of the time. Many people did not have enough to eat themselves, yet spontaneously shared what they had with the workers. The contribution of time and resources to collective projects was seen as demonstrative of meaningful participation of the community in the overall intervention. While some organizations, such as the CDR, in the affected neighborhoods were criticized for not doing enough, the FMC was recognized and praised for the work they did, and specifically for creating new mechanisms to enhance participation, as noted below.

Workshops conducted to take stock of Plan Cayo Hueso underscored the strong feeling held that while the interventions had contributed positively and had succeeded in stimulating activity and involvement in the community ("this was more than a construction project . . ."), the need to improve the conditions of those most in need still persisted. In this regard, specific attention was given to the capacities for meeting such challenges and to the ways in which Plan Cayo Hueso had contributed.

Dengue: Crisis and Prevention

In 2001 to 2002, Havana was threatened by a serious outbreak of dengue fever, a mosquito-borne disease that had been raging in the Latin American and Caribbean region and worldwide since the late 1990s (Gubler, 2005). Widespread mobilization of people and resources to isolate cases, intensely fumigate, and eliminate actual and potential mosquito-breeding sites were remarkably successful in limiting what could have been a very serious health impact, and earned much recognition worldwide (Spiegel et al., 2002). Nevertheless, the experience drew attention to the need for improving the methods that could be pursued to prevent and control this disease.

This section explains how an integrated approach was undertaken to manage dengue by focusing on both responding to the crisis and moving beyond it to achieve sustainability.

Because no vaccine for dengue fever exists, health protection has emphasized the prevention and control of urban cycles of *Aedes aegypti* mosquito-to-human transmission. Increased attention has been given to the application of an integrated approach to overcome barriers and establish bridges to sustainable management (Spiegel et al., 2005). The challenges to achieving this were formidable, as coordination was required across a wide range of organizations that otherwise tend to act quite independently of one another.

While epidemics of dengue-like virus were well known in Cuba prior to 1945, for almost three decades until the late 1970s there was no recognized disease presence in Cuba and across the countries of the Western Hemisphere because of the widespread use of pesticides such as DDT (Gubler & Clark, 1996). Nevertheless, in 1977, after it was officially declared that *Aedes aegypti* had been eliminated in Cuba, the country experienced its first nationwide dengue epidemic of "modern times." In 1981, an explosive epidemic due to a different strain struck the island, producing the first appearance of dengue haemorrhagic fever (DHF) in the Americas. It was also countrywide in Cuba, with approximately 344,203 dengue fever cases, more than 10,000 DHF cases, and 158 deaths (Guzman, Kouri, Bravo, et al., 1990).

Dengue Control in Cuba

Cuba's present-day mosquito control program was initiated during the 1981 DHF epidemic and characterized then by a vertically structured (top-down) mosquito-control emphasis (Gubler & Clark, 1996). While the design strategy applied in Cuba was in many ways similar to that nominally identified in other countries, the intensity and comprehensiveness of implementation was quite distinct. Unlike with other countries that had tended to disband their dengue-control activities over the 1980s and 1990s, when dengue reemerged in the Latin American and Caribbean region, Cuba's comprehensive public-health infrastructure to control DHF still existed in Cuba.

On a regular cycle of approximately twice a month, a team of inspectors (known as *campañistas* or *operarios*) checked houses for the presence of breeding sites and the presence of unhygienic conditions, giving fines for poor sanitation practices. The comprehensive primary-care network available for diagnosis and treatment of health concerns was further complemented by the internationally recognized expertise in vector-borne disease of the Pedro Kouri Institute for Tropical Medicine (IPK). This structure for disease prevention continues today.

During the 2001 to 2002 epidemic, the government of Cuba trained and mobilized an additional fifteen thousand workers to go from house to house to implement mosquito control and educate citizens about dengue and control of *Aedes aegypti* mosquitoes. Massive amounts of insecticide were used for larval and adult mosquito control. Water containers were treated with larvicides, houses sprayed with residual insecticides, and weekly spraying was conducted both indoors and outdoors. Building on Cuba's strong history of effective public-health education, awareness campaigns were intensified. Elementary schools taught children on Saturdays how to clean the house and yard to prevent mosquito breeding grounds. Television programs provided basic education on potential health concerns and prevention strategies.

Although the emergency-response capacity proved to be strong, the costs and risks associated with facing crisis situations were deemed to be too great to just rely on this. Accordingly, the national government expressed a strong interest in providing greater health protection through a more comprehensive, integrated management of factors that could result in dengue outbreaks. In this context, a pilot project to create an integrated surveillance system for dengue control was undertaken in Central Havana through a research program in collaboration with the Canadian International Development Research Centre, building on the previous Cayo Hueso experience (Bonet et al., 2007).

The initiative undertaken featured three main subsystems and builds on existing strengths, but aims to improve on the relevance and timeliness of information available to achieve effective dengue control. The components include the following:

1. *Epidemiological clinical surveillance*—collecting and analyzing information on the individuals at risk, probable or confirmed cases, and serological surveillance;

2. *Entomological surveillance*—constituting active surveillance in the areas of infestation and appearance of epidemic foci; and

3. *Environmental surveillance*—allowing the identification and stratification of risks within each of the five people's councils of Central Havana (distinguishing the driving forces, pressures, and state indicators).

In addition, development and close monitoring of community participation is central to the program's success—at all times, not only during epidemics.

In a series of interviews conducted with decision makers in Central Havana, specific problems with the preexisting surveillance systems were identified, confirming the need to move to a more integrated approach. Environmental surveillance was identified as an area where improvement was especially required, given Central Havana's widely prevalent infrastructural problems in areas such as blocked drainage, construction debris, water leaks, and vacant lots. Flooded basements, inaccessible areas, water tanks in poor condition, and water leaks were also specifically mentioned as areas that required closer monitoring. Accordingly, these particular conditions were added to the indicators that would be systematically inspected and recorded by the *operarios* in their reports.

Decision makers also identified other factors, such as high turnover of personnel, lack of motivation, poor quality of inspection, and inadequately qualified staff, as organizational issues that could seriously undermine effective operation of the program itself. It was also thought that communication between family doctors and the *operarios* could be made more timely and systematic, and that mass organizations in the community such as the CDR and FMC could contribute much through more systematic involvement. Furthermore, there was irregular cross-communication between environmental and epidemiological surveillance. It was also acknowledged that despite educational campaigns during crisis periods, there remained limited action at the community level.

Capacity as a Social Network

The value of surveillance and predictive tools lies in the ability to implement effective intervention measures by providing decision makers with the information they need early on. Workshops to select a new set of indicators were held with the participation of all the organizations that would both provide and use the information in the integrated surveillance program. Additionally, the tracking form for the environmental inspectors was modified, and training sessions were held to prepare the *operarios*.

Through the systematic collection of data on the identified indicators, a comprehensive profile of trends and distribution of factors relevant to the incidence of dengue was assembled. Research was conducted to characterize the knowledge, attitudes, and behaviors of the local community and to identify the risk factors associated with the presence of breeding sites. This helped to better target further operation of the integrated surveillance networks and evaluate the linkage of the various agencies and community organizations.

Until a vaccine is successfully developed, an integrated, community-based program connected to different units that collect needed information remains the most critical way to reduce the incidence of dengue (Pan American Health Organization, 1995; 2001). Experience in communities such as Central Havana, and exploring ways to institutionalize links with government agencies, can provide the evidence base for practices and methods that can achieve sustainable prevention and control of this important health threat.

Tourism Expansion: Adapting to Growth

A key part of the Cuban government's response to the collapse of its Socialist bloc trading partners in the early 1990s was the decision to open the island to global tourism, in essence developing this industry into one of Cuba's most important economic activities.

Despite the promise of prosperity that is the allure of tourism expansion worldwide, there is growing evidence of a risk of negative impacts on the health and well-being of local populations (Apostolopoulos & Sonmez, 2002; Frechtling, 1997; Stonich, 1998). In Cuba, this presented a distinct challenge: On the one hand, while needed foreign exchange largely motivated tourism expansion, the uneven access to such funds by those involved in the tourism sector provided additional pressure on a society that "shared its poverty" relatively equally with a strongly integrated equity in the provision of goods and services for its citizens. On the other hand, the unique Cuban context provided an interesting response to such threats and opportunities, especially in comparison to how this is addressed in other low- and middle-income countries.

Responding to Potential Impacts

As the effects of tourism are most intensely felt at a local level, it is especially instructive to consider how communities respond to such change. To do this, our Canadian-Cuban research team established a partnership with two distinct coastal communities: Caibarién, a community that is at the early stages of tourism development; and Cárdenas, a community with a long history of tourism involvement (Figure 10.1).

Caibarién is a fishing town of forty thousand, connected by a newly constructed, 80-kilometer causeway (only partially completed at the time of the study) to the new tourism destination in the North-East Keys of Villa Clara Province. Cárdenas is a city with a population of approximately a hundred thousand that is adjacent to the well-established resort destination of Varadero and is home to the majority of tourism

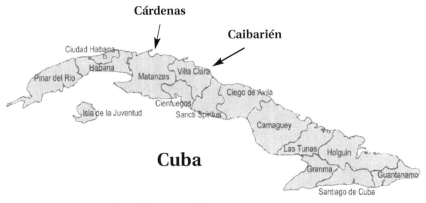

FIGURE 10.1 *Tourism Study Communities*

workers in this region. Focus groups were held in each community, each grouping individuals with distinct relations to tourism development: (a) decision makers (representing government and city officials); (b) community members (members of the community at large, including farmers, workers, teachers); (c) health-related workers; and (d) tourism-industry workers. In addition, key informant interviews were held.

Based on the information that emerged, health concerns were grouped in the following areas: psychosocial concerns, occupational health, infectious and chronic diseases, and societal and environmental concerns. Finally, community meetings were held to report on the findings and identify areas felt to be of particular concern for future policy and action. All focus-group participants and key informants were invited to attend these meetings. This provided a space for reflection, as well as an opportunity to take stock of existing processes underway.

All focus groups noted that "tourism has a physical and psychological impact on people," (see Table 10.1) and both communities raised numerous health concerns. These included psychosocial factors (changing values, disparity, dysfunctional families, and mental health stress related to "prominent [economic] difference between the workers in tourism and the rest of the community"); occupational health impacts (job-related stress, gender-specific factors such as work extending "well into pregnancy," and toxic exposures); infectious and chronic diseases (e.g., HIV/AIDS); broader societal impacts (e.g., prostitution); and environmental effects (e.g., waste).

Most significant, a wide range of programs were seen to have been established in the communities to mitigate potentially negative impacts of tourism, as summarized in Table 10.2. Some of the programs were local adaptations of national programs (e.g., *Barrio Debate* [Neighborhood Debates], which in these communities focused on tourism expan-

Table 10.1   Tourism Impacts Identified by Focus Groups

Focus groups Communities	Decision makers Cárdenas	Decision makers Caibarién	Community Cárdenas	Community Caibarién	Health Cárdenas	Health Caibarién	Tourism Cárdenas	Tourism Caibarién
Psychosocial								
Mental health	●							
Changing values/lifestyle			●	●		●	●	●
Social/econ disparity	●	●	●	●				●
Dysfunctional families	●	⊙	●			●	●	●
Alcoholism		●			●	●		
Tobacco use					●			
Drug addiction	●		●					⊙
Obesity					●	●		
Occupational health								
Job stress/pressure	●				●	●	●	●
Physical strain/demands	●				●	●	●	●
Exposure to toxic agents					●			
Infectious and chronic diseases								
STIs (HIV/AIDS)	●				●	●		⊙
VBDs				⊙	⊙	⊙		
Food poisoning					●	●		
Cardio, cerebrovascular					●	●		
Societal								
Corruption and unlawful activities	●		●					
Tourist harassment			●					●
Traffic-related accidents					●			
Prostitution	●		●	⊙				⊙
Need larger hospital			●	●				
Environmental								
Waste-related		●	●	●				
Other ecological (pollution, toxic waste)			●	⊙		●	●	

●: Issue identified as being experienced.   ⊙: Issue identified as an area of concern/anticipation.
Source: Spiegel et al., 2008a.

sion). Through this program, for example, a new waste-management system for the community was established in Cárdenas, and one physician was placed in each resort hotel. Group members noted that all types of concerns could be voiced at these meetings, and thus the group, while sponsoring direct mitigation efforts, was indirectly creating stronger social cohesion and reducing mental stress.

In response to increased alcoholism and drug abuse, focus-group members in Caibarién observed that the municipal authority had developed two radio programs that aired each week for one hour. The aim of both programs was to promote health education while emphasizing the risks of alcoholism and drug abuse. The radio programs were thought to be specifically targeted toward at-risk populations such as those working within the tourism industry or youth prone to alcohol and drug use due to increased exposure to tourism.

Table 10.2   Mitigating Programs and Areas of Coverage Reported by Focus Groups

Caibarién

Mitigating program or strategy	Area of concern	Focus
Project management office in the People's Power people's council in 2000	Impact of tourism; health promotion *National policy*	Community capacity; youth; tourism projects
Radio programs	General health; drug and alcohol addiction	Youth; family; community; tourism workers; health education
Pamphlet distribution	Drug and alcohol; STIs; use of condoms *Through the Provincial Center of Hygiene and Epidemiology*	Population in general and tourists
Barrio Debate	Any community concern; social cohesion; psychosocial effects of tourism *National project*	All community members
Art show	HIV/AIDS	Public in general; community
Media displays in schools	HIV/AIDS	All students; youth
Community health programs	STIs; health risks; prostitution; alcohol, tobacco, and drug addiction; sexuality; birth control	Tourism workers; students; school counselors
Reunión del sistema	Community well-being; vector surveillance; intersectoral decision making	Community as a whole; professionals in different sectors
Jardines del Rey	Sanitation in the community; waste management; environment *Other jurisdiction in Cuba Model for Caibarién*	Public in general in resort community
Mi casa bonita, mi casa saludable	Sanitation at home and surrounding environment	Householders
Deployment of physicians with specialty in Work Medicine in resorts	Health promotion; prevention of diseases; vector control *National program*	Tourists; tourism workers
Deployment of social workers: Happy Youth Project	Psychosocial health; mental-health promotion	Youth; families
Alvaro Reinoso Task in the tourism workers neighborhood of Van Troy	Problem identification through focus groups *National program*	Displaced workers; tourism workers; community

Cárdenas

Mitigating program or strategy	Area of concern	Focus
Project management office in the People's Power people's council in 2000	Impact of tourism; health promotion *National policy*	Community capacity; youth; tourism projects
Actions for the creation of positive tourism	Harassment of tourists; mental health; corruption and other crime	Youth; community capacity building
Popular Shield	Drug and alcohol addiction *National program*	Tourism students; youth education; at-risk youth; tourists
Committee for Transit Safety	Motor vehicle accidents and road safety	Public in general; tourists
Deployment of physicians with specialty in Work Medicine in resorts	Health promotion; prevention of diseases; vector control *National program*	Tourists; tourism workers
Local government committees such as: Committee against drugs Committee against STIs	STIs; promotion of safe sex; addictions; road safety; housing for tourists	Community as a whole in its different aspects
Student Volunteer Brigades	Sanitation; environment	Cleaning beaches and surroundings
Research projects	Impacts of tourism on society and environment	Decision makers at municipal level

Source: Spiegel et al., 2008a.

Promotional and literacy pamphlets, developed in conjunction with the Provincial Center of Hygiene and Epidemiology, also outlined the risks of alcohol and drug consumption and sexually transmitted illnesses (STIs), and promoted the use of condoms. Industry workers helped distribute the pamphlets in hotels and at local restaurants. Similarly, community-health programming targeted tourism workers, students, and school counselors through the distribution of educational material dealing with the health risks involved in prostitution, alcoholism, and tobacco and drug use. It was noted that this educational material was available at tourism-training institutes as well. In addition, community health workers reported visits to local schools in an effort to encourage discussion with students and school counselors in these areas. All the above efforts were financially supported by the Cuban government. Furthermore, local government committees existed to address problematic areas of STIs, addictions, safety, and housing for tourists.

Besides targeting specific public-health areas or population groups, intersectoral coordination across areas of concern and within multiple sectors of the community were noted. In Caibarién, *Reunión del Sistema* [System Meetings] were held weekly involving health-care professionals and community leaders from various sectors and levels of government. At these sessions, the issue of vector surveillance was routinely examined and decisions were made regarding health interventions and interventions for community well-being in general.

In response to increased social pressures, a program in Cárdenas known as *Acciones para la Creación del Turismo Positivo* [Actions for the Creation of Positive Tourism] has offered youth events such as arts, crafts, sport, and dance twice weekly. It was felt that this sort of activity would improve the mental well-being and coping mechanisms of youth participants. In addition, Cárdenas was noted to have employed community workers to advertise this youth program within the community, at the beaches in particular, and in so doing increased community capacity to respond to health concerns. All events arranged for the youth were free, funded in part by municipal authorities and in part by local resorts as a "pay back or compensation" to local communities. Student Volunteer Brigades were reported to have been periodically dispatched to clean beaches and surrounding areas.

Capacity to Respond to Global Forces

The variety of programs identified in the two Cuban communities studied shows creativity and a strong commitment to address the impacts of tourism. Although the results of such efforts cannot yet be determined, the efforts implemented by local communities have been seen by community members as positive. Moreover, this case study of two communities in Cuba illustrated that communities can and do create programs and improve infrastructure to sustain population health not only in reaction to pressures, but in anticipation of change. The widespread global phenomenon of comparable tourism expansion thus sets out an interesting context for comparative analysis with other countries.

Lessons from the Cuban Experience

The case studies discussed above illustrate how local health-service providers, sectors with responsibilities for factors that can affect health, local government, and members of affected communities in Cuba have systematically been able to interact at a community level to address health concerns. These processes, which resemble the kind of intersectoral collaborations proposed by the Alma-Ata recommendations, are especially notable in comparison to the weakening of public-sector structures affecting most other low- and middle-income countries. Rather than consider this an exotic Cuban phenomenon, it is valuable to reflect on two key attributes that can be discerned from this variation:

1. That the capacity to collectively engage different social forces to address health concerns is perhaps a more appropriate consideration of the construct of "social capital" than seen in many other countries; and

2. That "political will" as an expression of policy orientation and commitment is ultimately of critical importance, and observable at different highly relevant points.

Social Capital

In the context of Western social science's discourse that is ideologically strongly focused on individualism and the health of individuals, "social capital" has been widely regarded as ". . . those features of social organization such as networks of secondary associations, high levels of interpersonal trust and norms of mutual aid and reciprocity which act as resources for individuals and facilitate collective action" (Lochner, Kawachi, & Kennedy, 1999, p. 260). The notion of social capital as a resource for communities, however, has been repeatedly observed in diverse settings to be associated with positive health in contrast to contexts that focus on the attributes of individuals (i.e., it is more beneficial to live in a place with high trust and connectivity than to have these attributes personally). Indeed, in our research in Cayo Hueso, we observed that the association of high self-rated health was greater for individuals living in neighborhoods marked by high degrees of trust and social connections than for those who personally had these attributes relative to others but were living in less "connected" communities.

However, just as posing the question of what makes some people healthy and others not tends to call into question the effect of determinants on health *within* a society, examining variation at the level of different forms of social organization, it may also call into question the effect variations in social cohesion that can be observed *among* different societies. This relates well to the observations that equity and power (and state role) need more attention (Sapag & Kawashi, 2007) and that power and inequities need to become more central to the analysis of social capital and not just regarded as "confounding variables" (Fine, 2001).

As the Alma-Ata declaration itself suggests, in order to achieve "health for all" it is necessary that greater integration in the interaction of social forces be pursued. Witnessing the development of greater intersectoral involvement and community engagement, our research team has been more drawn to consider the policy relevance of "community capacity" as a relevant expression of social capital.

Just as other forms of capital refer to resources that may be harnessed to facilitate the pursuit of a common enterprise (e.g., economic capital referring to economic assets that can be applied), social capital can be seen to be the capacity to actively engage social actors to undertake common purpose, such as the social production of health. In this sense, social capital can be seen to be observable in three dimensions of what may be called community capacity:

1. Credible *infrastructure* and *resources* that are locally available to address population health and its determinants;

2. Capacity to work *together* to effectively address determinants; and

3. A *space for community and citizen involvement* in setting the agenda and being actively involved in addressing issues of concern.

The Cuban experience, as illustrated in the case study discussions, demonstrates that these three attributes have been strongly and systematically present and engaged. In this sense, there is good reason to think that these constructs should be considered further in comparative analyses as key elements of social capital that can have great policy relevance for improving population health.

Political Will

The elephant in the room in discussions of how and where progress in population health was achieved following Alma-Ata has been political systems. Cuba not only achieved health breakthroughs immediately following its revolution, it has sustained them amid great economic difficulties. Discussion with our Cuban colleagues on the social production of health and the management of health determinants inevitably turns to a discussion of political will. And in Western capitalist societies, the degree to which health concerns are addressed and make it to an agenda is no less important. In short, policy matters!

While political will does not by itself produce positive health outcomes, it undeniably has a critical role in determining how the resources and organization needed to produce positive health outcomes can be engaged and applied. In this sense, it can be observed in its expression of commitment and evaluated in its implementation.

A common metric used as an expression of political will is the percentage of budget allocated to health. But this is at best very limited, and at worst a caricature that can recognize inefficiencies as beneficial. In this sense, the form of evaluation applied to industrial enterprises provides a useful framework to use, focusing on structure, process, and output. In the Cuban context, the commitment to forms of organization that are inclusive of health concerns, the maintenance of basic health-system infrastructure, and the allocation of stable budgets amid competing priorities are expressions of political will.

Conclusions

In light of the observation of how health determinants have been addressed, as well as health services organized, the Cuban paradox (How can a poor country produce good health results?) tends to become more comprehensible. There is, after all, very little paradox in having good health produced in a country that systematically has organized its priorities in this direction by actually applying the principles of Alma-Ata. The paradox, perhaps, is how we could think otherwise.

References

Apostolopoulos, Y., & Sonmez, S. (2002). Disease mapping and risk assessment for public health and sustainable tourism development in insular regions. In J. Gayle (Ed.), *Island tourism and sustainable development* (pp. 225–248). Westport, CT: Praeger Publishers.

Bonet M., Spiegel J., Ibarra, A. M., Kouri, G., Pintre, A., & Yassi, A. (2007). An integrated ecosystem approach for sustainable prevention and control of dengue in Central Havana. *International Journal of Occupational and Environmental Health, 13*(2), 188–194.

Breman, A., & Shelton, C. (2001). *Structural adjustment and health: A literature review of the debate, its role players and presented empirical evidence* (draft for discussion). World Health Organization: Commission on Macroeconomics and Health, Paper WG6: June 6, 2001.

Brown, T. M., Cueto, M., & Fee, E. (2006). The World Health Organization and the transition from "international" to "global" public health. *American Journal of Public Health, 96*, 62–72.

Castell, F. P. (2007*). La intersectorialidad en la practica social.* La Habana, Cuba: Editorial Ciencias Medicas.

Castro Ruiz, F. Address by Dr. Fidel Castro Ruz, president of the Council of State and the Council of Ministers of the Republic of Cuba. In the Group of 77 South Summit Conference, April 12, 2000, Havana. Retrieved May 23, 2008, from http://www.granma.cu/documento/ingles00/009-i.html

Chappotin, A. S. (1998). El taller de transformación integral: una alternativa más de desarrollo comunitario en Cuba. In R. Dávalos (Ed.), *Desarrollo local y descentralización en el contexto urbano.* Vol. III. Universidad de La Habana, Cuba.

Commission on Social Determinants of Health. (2007). Interim Report. *Achieving health equity: From root causes to fair outcomes.* World Health Organization, Geneva. Available online at http://whqlibdoc.who.int/publications/2007/interim_statement_eng.pdf

Commission on Social Determinants of Health. (2008). *Closing the gap in a generation: Health equity through action on the social determinants of health.* World Health Organization, Geneva. Available online at http://www.who.int/social_determinants/final_report/en/index.html

Coyula, M., & Hamberg, J. (2003). The case of Havana, Cuba. In *Understanding slums: Case studies for the global report 2003,* UN HABITAT. Available at http://www.ucl.ac.uk/dpu-projects/Global_Report/pdfs/Havana.pdf

de la Torre, E., Márquez, M., Gutiérrez Muñiz, J.A., López Pardo, C., & Rojas Ochoa, F. (2004). *La salud para todos sí es posible.* Havana, Cuba: Sociedad Cubana de Salud Pública.

Dilla, H., & Oxhorn, P. (2002).The virtues and misfortunes of civil society in Cuba. *Latin American Perspectives, 29*, 11–30.

Dollar, D. (2001). Is globalization good for your health? *WHO Bulletin, 79*(9), 827–833.

Dollar, D., & Kraay A. (2002). Growth is good for the poor. *Journal of Economic Growth, 7*, 195–225.

Feinsilver, J. (1993). *Healing the masses: Cuban health politics at home and abroad.* Berkeley, CA: University of California Press.

Field, C. [Director and Producer], Bourne, Keck, & Reed [Producers]. (2006). *Salud!* [documentary film]. Cuba.

Fine, B. (2001). *Social capital versus social theory.* London; Routledge.

Frechtling, D. C. (1997). Current research on health and tourism issues and future directions. In S. Clift & P. Grabowski (Eds.), *Tourism and health: Risks, research and responses.* Washington DC: Pinter Press.

Garfield, R., & Santana, S. (1997). The impact of the economic crisis and the US embargo on health in Cuba. *American Journal of Public Health*, January, 87(1), 15–20.

Gubler, D. J. (2005). The emergence of epidemic dengue fever and dengue hemorrhagic fever in the Americas: A case of failed public health policy. *Pan American Journal of Public Health*, 17(4), 221–224.

Gubler, D. J., & Clark, G. G. (1996). Community involvement in the control of *Aedes aegypti*. *Acta Tropica*, 61, 169–179.

Guzman M. G., Kouri G., Bravo J., et al. (1990). Dengue hemorrhagic fever in Cuba, 1981: A retrospective seroepidemiologic study. *American Journal of Tropical Medicine and Hygiene*, 429(2), 179–184.

Harvey, D. (2005). *A brief history of neoliberalism*. New York: Oxford University Press.

INHEM (1999). Instituto Nacional De Higiene, Epidemiología y Microbiología, Centro Colaborador de la OMS en el Área de Salud de la Vivienda. *Plan de medidas ejecutadas por el gobierno y la comunidad (PMGC) en Cayo Hueso*, 1996–1999, Havana, Cuba.

Kirkpatrick, A. F. (1997). The US attack on Cuba's health. *Canadian Medical Association Journal*, 157, 281–284.

Labonte, R., & Schrecker, T. (2007). Foreign policy matters; a normative view of the G8 and population health. *Globalization and Health*, 3, 7.

Lochner, K., Kawachi I., &, Kennedy, B. P. (1999). Social capital: A guide to its measurement. *Health and Place*, 5(4), 259–270.

Macdonald, T. (1985). *Making a new people: Education in revolutionary Cuba*. Vancouver: New Star Books, Ltd.

MacDonald, T. (1999). A Developmental analysis of Cuba's health care system since 1959. *Studies in Health and Human Services (Vol. 32)*. Lewiston, NY: Edwin Mellen Press.

Maciocco, G., et al. (2008). From Alma Ata to the Global Fund: The history of international health policy. Prepared by the Italian Global Health Watch. *Social Medicine*, 3(1), 36–48.

Pan American Health Organization. (1995). Dengue y dengue hemorrágico en las Américas: Guías para su prevencion y control. Scientific publication No. 548. Washington, DC: PAHO.

Pan American Health Organization (2001). Dengue prevention and control Resolution CE 128. R3 of the 43rd Directing Council of the Pan American Health Organization. Washington, DC: PAHO.

Roman, P. (1999). *People's power. Cuba's experience with representative government*. Boulder, CO: Westview Press.

Sapag, J. C., & Kawachi, I. (2007). Social capital and health promotion in Latin America. *Journal of Public Health*, 41(1), 139–149.

Schwab, P. (1999). *Cuba: Confronting the U.S. embargo*. New York: St. Martin's Press.

Spiegel, J. M., Bennett, S., Hattersley, L., et al. (2005). Barriers and bridges to prevention and control of dengue: The need for a social-ecological approach. *EcoHealth*, 2(4), 273–290.

Spiegel, J. M., Bonet, M., Yassi, A., Molina, E., Concepción, M. & Mas, P. (2001). Developing ecosystem health indicators in Centro Habana: A community-based approach. *Ecosystem Health*, 7(1), 15–26.

Spiegel, J., Bonet, M., Yassi, A., Tate, R. B., Concepción, M., & Canizares, M. (2003). Evaluating the effectiveness of a multi-component intervention to improve health in an inner-city Havana Community. *International Journal of Environmental and Occupational Health, 9*(2), 118–127.

Spiegel, J. M., Garcia, M., Yassi, A., & Bonet, M. (2005). Learning together: A Canada-Cuba research collaboration to improve the sustainable management of environmental health risks. *Canadian Journal of Public Health, 97*(1).

Spiegel, J. M., Gonzalez, M., Cabrera, G. J., Catasus, S., Vidal, C., Yassi A. (2008a). Promoting health in response to global tourism expansion in Cuba. *Health Promotion International, 23*, 60–69.

Spiegel, J. M., Yassi, A., & Tate, R. (2002). Dengue in Cuba: Mobilization against Aedes aegypti. *Lancet Infectious Disease, 2*, 204–205.

Spiegel, J. M., & Yassi, A. (2004). Lessons from the margins of globalization: Appreciating the Cuban health paradox. *Journal of Public Health Policy, 25*, 85–110.

Spiegel, J. M., Bonet, M., Alvarez, A., Castel-Floret, P., & Millar, J. (2008b). *Intersectorality in the social production of health: Sharing perspectives and experiences to orient a Cuba-Canada research program.* Workshop Proceedings. February 17–19, 2008, Havana, Cuba. http://www.ligi.ubc.ca/?p2=/modules/liu/researches/category.jsp&id=25

Stonich, S. (1998). Political ecology of tourism. *Annals of Tourism Research, 25*, 5–54.

Tate, R. B., Fernandez, N., Yassi, A., Canizare, M., Spiegel, J. M., & Bonet, M. (2003). Change in health risk perception following community intervention in Central Havana, Cuba. *Health Promotion International, 18*(4), 279–286.

Whiteford, L. M., & Branch, L. G. (2008). *Primary health care in Cuba: The other revolution.* Lanham, MD: Rowman & Littlefield.

WHO-UNICEF. (1978). Alma-Ata Declaration. *Primary health care.* Health for All Series Number 1. Geneva, World Health Organization.

World Bank. (1993). Investing in Health. *World development report.* New York: Oxford University Press.

World Health Organization. (2003). *Macroeconomics and health: Investing in health for economic development.* Geneva: World Health Organization.

Yassi, A., Mas, P., Bonet, M., Tate, R., Fernandez, N., & Spiegel, J. (1999). Applying an ecosystem approach to the determinants of health in Centro Habana. *Ecosystem Health, 5*, 3–19.

Yassi, A., et al. (2003). Community participation in a multi-sectoral intervention to address health determinants in an inner city community in Central Havana. *Journal of Urban Health, 80*, 61–80.

Young, A. H. (1985). *Comparative urbanization.* New Orleans, LA: University of New Orleans.

PART III

Social Services and Health Care

CHAPTER ELEVEN

Social Work and Health Care

David L. Strug
Odalys González Jubán

Social workers have played an important role in the Cuban health-care system since the early days of the revolution. Shortly after the triumph of the revolution in 1959, the government determined that Cuba needed trained social workers to assist health-care professionals in bolstering the country's public-health infrastructure, which had deteriorated considerably owing to the emigration of large numbers of health professionals (Bravo, 1998).

In 1971, the Cuban Ministry of Public Health (MINSAP) established special schools to train social workers in health care to assist doctors, nurses, and other health-care professionals in hospitals and medical clinics throughout the country. Almost all of Cuba's social workers in health care were trained at schools that functioned until the end of the 1990s. Starting in 2003, MINSAP acknowledged the important role social workers play in the health-care system by initiating a social and occupational rehabilitation program leading to a *Licenciatura* degree (roughly equivalent to a master's degree in social work), which is offered by the Advanced Institute of Medical Sciences (*Instituto Superior de Ciencias Médicas*) in Havana. The goal of this program is to train social workers to assist individuals with different levels of temporary or chronic disability in need of physical rehabilitation and psychosocial readjustment.

MINSAP employs more social workers than any other government department. Most health social workers in Cuba are members of the Society of Cuban Social Workers in Health Care, the only professional social work organization in the country. The government recognizes the important consultative, educational, and organizational functions of this organization, which it supports by funding educational and training seminars for its members at the provincial, municipal, and national levels. The organization's scientific committee sponsors an international social work conference every two years with the assistance of MINSAP officials, which is attended by social workers from all over Latin America and other parts of the world.

Social workers in the health field collaborate closely with other health-care professionals and operate at all levels of the national health-care system in both urban and rural areas. Hospitals and polyclinics employ social workers to work with pregnant mothers, cancer patients, the elderly, the disabled, and a variety of other at-risk populations. Social workers are also employed at community mental-health programs and at HIV/AIDS prevention and treatment programs. They collaborate with family doctor/nurse teams in the community. The chapter on the frail elderly in this volume (chapter 13) describes the close working relationship of a polyclinic social worker and a family doctor with older community members. The Basic Work Group, an interdisciplinary team that provides consultancy to the community-based family doctor/nurse team, typically has a social worker as part of its group.

The following interview that one of the editors (David Strug) conducted with Odalys González Jubán, the president of the Cuban Society of Social Workers in Health Care and a practicing social worker at a municipal polyclinic in Havana, illustrates how social workers in health care collaborate in an interdisciplinary fashion and work in an intersectorial context at all levels of the national health care system. It also describes González Jubán's view of what makes social work in Cuba different from social work in other countries as well as her perspective on how social work in health care on the island mirrors the values of the Cuban Revolution. This interview underscores her pride in being a health social worker in Cuba.

González Jubán, like most social workers in health care in Cuba, received her training in social work and health at a specialized technical training institute for social workers rather than at a university. These training institutes no longer exist in the country. Social workers in health care were until recently viewed as technicians rather than health-care professionals like doctors and nurses, and it was not considered necessary to graduate from a university to become a social work technician, as was true in Odalys's case (Strug, 2006).

An Interview with Odalys González Jubán, Havana, Cuba, December, 2007

O.G.J. My name is Odalys González Jubán and I was born in the city of Havana on May 29, 1963. I graduated from middle school and then majored in social work in high school. In 2004, I began a *licenciatura* degree program (roughly equivalent to a master's degree in the U.S.) specializing in social and occupational rehabilitation, and I should be finishing up with this program in July 2008.* This program combines social work and occupational therapy.

D.S.   *Why did you choose social work as a profession?*

O.G.J. Really, in some sense it was my mother who chose it for me. "You will learn a lot about people's needs and problems and you will be able to help them," she said to me. I think my interest in social work really goes back to my grandmother who, although not having any formal knowledge about social work, was nevertheless a true social worker. She helped out her neighbors, and she took in and raised two children who were not part of our family. So everything I have done in social work is based on the values of cooperation, solidarity, and altruism, which I think I got from my grandmother through our family bloodline. I knew little about what social work was at the beginning of my education. But when I started studying social work, I fell in love with the profession. It is a beautiful career, of great help to people, and these are the qualities that I recognize as important to me. So I liked the career a great deal. I have tried all I can as president of the Society of Social Workers in Health Care to advance the profession of social work because of the love I have for this type of work.

D.S.   *Do you think if there had been no Cuban Revolution you would have become a social worker?*

O.G.J. I think so. Social work gives me so much personally. It gives me knowledge and the ability to understand people and to imagine myself in their situation. Even when I can't necessarily offer clients material help, at least I can help them spiritually by listening to them talk about their problems. This listening and helping is also a form of healing ourselves as social workers.

---

* Odalys González Jubán finished this program in July 2008 and will be working on her doctorate starting in 2009.

D.S.   *Besides being the president of the Society of Social Workers in Health Care, you work in a polyclinic. What's that work like?*

O.G.J.   The polyclinic offers primary health care to community members. I work with people who have social problems related to their health status. My work also involves helping clients get free medicine, assisting women who are breastfeeding, helping pregnant mothers who are socially disadvantaged, assisting patients with mental-health problems, and aiding older persons get the services they need. I am part of the mental-health commission within our polyclinic, and I work with different types of interdisciplinary and intersectorial organizations, which the *Consejo Popular*† brings together.

D.S.   *What relationship do you have with the Consejo Popular?*

O.G.J.   There is a direct connection between the polyclinic and the *Consejo Popular*. The *Consejo Popular* is comprised of a number of commissions of different organizations that include representatives of mass organizations, community representatives, directors of state enterprises, and other individuals. The director of our polyclinic is a member of the *Consejo Popular*. A Commission for Social Prevention (*Comisión de Prevención y Atención Social*) also forms part of the *Consejo Popular*. This commission addresses social problems at the local level, like cases of delinquency or alcoholism. As the social worker of my polyclinic, I participate alongside representatives of mass organizations, community leaders, and other members of this committee in an effort to resolve problems in the community, especially those problems that are related to health and illness.

D.S.   *What would you say is unique about Cuban social work, given your international experience in the social work profession?*

O.G.J.   Social work is different in each country; social work in Cuba and elsewhere reflects the political will of government to support or not support efforts to address social problems. Despite the fact that Cuba is a blockaded country, we attempt through the implementation of social policies to find alternative ways

---

† A *Consejo Popular*, or Popular Council, is a local entity comprised of community delegates and representatives of grassroots organizations, state enterprises, and administrative entities. It is a vehicle for decision making about meeting the economic, health, and social needs of community members under its jurisdiction (Roman, 2003).

of providing help for our citizens in need, although sometimes we may not have all the material resources for doing so.

The interdisciplinary and the intersectorial aspects of Cuban social work also distinguish social work in this country from social work elsewhere. We work as members of interdisciplinary teams and with other state entities and mass organizations, with considerable support from our political leaders. Our leaders programmatically direct our efforts to assist people in need of help.

Social work in Cuba is not a unified profession. Social workers are employed in a fragmented fashion in different state organizations and entities. It would be ideal if there were a single, more unified social work in Cuba where social workers were prepared to intervene in whatever type of situation.

D.S.   *What do you wish other countries might learn from Cuban social work?*

For me, social work is love, commitment, altruism, solidarity, brotherhood—and these are the values that I think social workers everywhere should incorporate. Not everyone can be a social worker. You have to carry this profession within your heart. I think the values of a good social worker in our country are also connected with the values of the Cuban Revolution, that is, they are the values of solidarity, respect, brotherhood, and altruism.

References

Bravo, E. M. (1998). *Development within underdevelopment: New trends in Cuban medicine*. Habana, Cuba: Editorial José Martí.

Roman, P. (2003). *People's power: Cuba's experience with representative government*. Lanham, MD: Rowman and Littlefield.

Strug, D. (2006). Community-oriented social work in Cuba: Government response to emerging social problems. *Social Work Education, 25*(7), 749–763.

CHAPTER TWELVE

Caring for People with Dementia in Cuba

Wendy Hulko
Niurka Cascudo Barral

One of the markers of the success of the Cuban Revolution is a life expectancy rate equal to that of developed countries. With this increase in the older population, Cuba is also seeing a rise in the number of people living with Alzheimer's disease (AD) and other forms of dementia. However, the care of people with dementia in Cuba does not mirror that of the global North or in developed countries: Cuban care is not as heavily dominated by bio-medicine and appears to be more holistic and community oriented.

This chapter addresses caring for community-dwelling older adults with dementia in Cuba. It starts with an overview of Cuba as an aging society, describes dementia in developing countries, and then proceeds with a discussion of primary health care in Cuba in general, and, more specifically, integrated care in the community for older adults. Next, there is a description of multidisciplinary gerontological care teams (EMAG) followed by a case study of an older Afro-Cuban woman with dementia. The chapter concludes with an analysis of Cuban approaches to dementia care in the form of reflections from the two coauthors: a Cuban doctor (Cascudo Barral) and a Canadian dementia researcher (Hulko).

Cuba as an Aging Society

Societal aging is a new phenomenon that has been the focus of concerted attention and vigorous debate in many countries of the North, particularly in North America and Western Europe. Population aging has been largely overlooked in the global South, however, as developing countries tend also to have a large proportion of children (Brink, 1997), and the growth of the older adult population has happened more recently and more rapidly than in the North (Ebrahim, 2002). Due to rapid technological advances in the 20th century, more and more people are living past eighty years of age (Harwood, Hirschfeld, & Sayer, 2004). Latin America and the Caribbean as a region is set to experience population aging at a fast pace, with the percentage of older people (sixty and older) projected to grow between 8 to 14 percent by 2025 (Albala et al., 2005). Within this region, a particular group of countries— Uruguay, Argentina, Cuba, and several countries in the Caribbean (Dutch Antilles, Guadalupe, Barbados, Martinique, and Puerto Rico)— are rapidly aging (CEPAL, 2003). In Cuba, the percentage of the population age sixty and older has grown from 9.1 percent in 1970 to 13.6 percent in 1998 (Gondor & Negrín, 1998) and currently sits at 15.9 percent (Oficina Nacional de Estadísticas [ONE], 2007).

Although Cuba has one of the fastest-aging populations in the developing world, there appears to be little research on aging in Cuba. In addition, it is doubtful whether findings from other parts of Latin America and the Caribbean can be generalized to Cuba, given that Cuba has less social stratification, higher education and literacy rates, and a universal, free public-health system (Herrera-Valdés & Almaguer-López, 2005), factors which make Cuba more comparable to developed than to developing countries. The limited research that exists on service design and delivery of care for older adults in Cuba reveals a variety of government programs developed since 1988 to improve the quality of life of older Cubans, to keep older Cubans engaged in society, and to teach youth that growing older is nothing to be ashamed of (Bertera, 2003; Strug, 2004). Many of the initiatives directed toward older adults are also available in developed countries; the difference, however, is that programs in Cuba are integrated into the community and rely on broad community support for their sustainability, moral exchanges, and reciprocities (Bertera, 2003; Strug, 2004).

Dementia in Developing Countries

There are multiple reasons why some older individuals develop dementia and others do not. Alzheimer's disease is the most common cause of dementia, especially among older adults with memory loss, lack of judgment, and disorientation (to time, place, and person being the key features) (Diamond, 2006). Numerous publications exist on the processes implicated in the normal aging of the brain and the differences that occur in Alzheimer's disease (AD) and other forms of cognitive impairment (Baggio et al., 1998; Diamond, 2006; Pliacentini et al., 2000; Robine & Vaupel, 2001). Some of the factors implicated in AD that have been investigated to date include oxidative mechanisms; genetic factors; environmental toxins; and illnesses such as ischemic cardiopathy, arterial hypertension, and diabetes mellitus (Martínez Lage, Hachinski, & Martínez Lage, 2001; Monti et al., 2000; National Institute on Aging, 2008; Ognibene et al., 1999; Wilson et al., 2002). Moreover, important studies in the United States (National Institute on Aging, 2007) and Canada (Lindsay et al., 2002) have revealed that lifestyle factors such as physical activity, a healthy diet, mentally stimulating activity, and social engagement can counterbalance a genetic bias toward developing this illness.

While "aging is not synonymous with infirmity," the aging of the population has resulted in a growth in the incidence of diseases associated with later life, such as Alzheimer's Disease. The relationship between AD and the aging process is well established: at the age of sixty-five, the risk of developing AD is 1 to 2 percent; and this figure doubles every five years to reach 30 to 32 percent at the age of eighty, after which the incidence begins to decrease (Florez-Tascón Sixto et al., 2003). The 10/66 Dementia Research Group, formed in 1998 to address the reality that "less than 10 percent of all population-based research into dementia is directed towards the two-thirds or more of cases living in developing parts of the world" (10/66 Dementia Research Group, 2000, p. 14), has conducted a number of incidence and prevalence studies on dementia in developing countries. The results indicate that 60.1 percent of all people living with dementia in 2001 were to be found in developing countries and that this number will increase to 64.5 percent in 2020 and 71.2 percent in 2040; further, the number of people with dementia in Latin America will nearly equal that of North America by 2040, despite being half the size at present (Ferri et al., 2005). In spite of a clear demographic imperative to shift our focus to the global South, knowledge of dementia in developing countries is largely limited to the work of the 10/66 Dementia Research Group, which to date has focused on incidence, prevalence, and risk factors (Ferri et al., 2005; Sánchez, 2006); culturally and educationally sensitive diagnoses (Prince, Acosta, Chui, Scazufca, & Varghese, 2003); and care arrangements (10/66 Dementia Research Group, 2004; Shaji, Smitha, Praveen, & Prince, 2003).

Studies of the Cuban population indicate that 4 to 5 percent of people over the age of sixty-five have dementia with a moderate degree of cognitive impairment, with the milder forms bringing the rates up to 10 percent (Carrasco, 2001; Hernández Pérez, 1999; Llibre Rodríguez & Hernández, 2002). Other research indicates that 10 percent of Cubans sixty-five years and older and 15 percent of Cubans over age eighty-five have dementia, which is similar to rates in developed countries like Spain (Navarra), where about ten thousand older adults have dementia (García, Rodríguez, & Jiménez, 2002). Cuban 10/66 researchers recently conducted a risk and prevalence study with 334 older adults (average age 76.5 years) in Havana and discovered prevalence rates of 3.8 percent for memory loss and 8.3 percent for dementia, the majority (twenty-five) of the cases being due to Alzheimer's and the remainder (five) being vascular in origin (Sánchez, 2006). The prevalence of dementia is similar to findings for Canada where 16 percent of people over the age of sixty-five have some degree of cognitive impairment and another 8 percent are diagnosed with Alzheimer's disease or another form of dementia (Canadian Institutes of Health Research [CIHR], 2007, p. 6; Canadian Study of Health and Aging [CSHA] Working Group, 1994).

Caring for people with dementia is costly, particularly in developing countries where social security and health services are minimal at best and nonexistent at worst (10/66 Dementia Research Group, 2004). Interviews with 706 people with dementia and their primary caregivers in India, China and South East Asia, Latin America, and the Caribbean (n=416), and Nigeria, led 10/66 researchers to the conclusion that caring for people with dementia in the developing world is "associated with substantial economic disadvantage" (10/66 Dementia Research Group, 2004, p. 175). However, this overall finding did not hold true for two of the study sites: Havana and Beijing, where there are universal and free public-health-care systems. In the developed world, dementia is the third most expensive disease in terms of social and economic costs, only preceded by cardiac disease and cancer, and places fourth among the principal causes of death in the older adult (Carrasco & Blas, 2004; De la Torre & Hachinski, 2002; Fillit & O'Concell, 2002, p. 211; Graff-Radford et al., 2007; Lussier, Malenfant, Peretz, & Beleville, 2001; Makoto Higuchi, 2005; Parkin, 2001).

The search for effective models of dementia care is driven in large part by a government's wish to reduce the costs associated with high use of health services by people with dementia and by the financial and psychological stresses experienced by family caregivers, who provide the majority of care for people with dementia (10/66 Dementia Research Group, 2004; Shaji et al., 2003). Health-care programs that are integrated into the community and deliver dementia care where persons with dementia and their families live are well poised to respond to this challenge. Not only can health-care providers establish the cognitive status of an older adult, they can assess other factors that are known to affect the health and quality of life of older adults as well. For example, the functional and cognitive status of older adults are markers of risk of development for dependency, institutionalization, caregiver stress and, more important, frailty and death (Kane, Ouslander, & Abrass, 2000). Therefore, in order to fully understand the care needs of older adults, as well as the interpersonal/intrafamilial conflicts and social problems present in their lives, primary health care in the community is the recommended approach.

Demographic Context of Primary Care in Cuba

Transformations in the ownership of private property and related social policies have been and continue to be the key focus of the Cuban Revolution (Saney, 2004). Since 1959, the principal objective of the economic system has been to achieve economic growth, while promoting equality and social justice. This has occurred through the construction of a society that upholds the principle of equal access to opportunities and in which the state is the guarantor of this objective (CEPDE, 2005).

The island of Cuba is going through a demographic process that is characterized by low levels of fertility and high survival rates, with more people every year reaching seventy-five years of age or more (Gondor & Negrín, 1998). By 2025, when one-quarter of the Cuban population will be sixty years of age and older, Cuba will be the "oldest country" in Latin America; and in 2050 not only will it be among the oldest in the world, but the population sixty years and older will be proportionally higher than that of half of all countries considered developed (CEPAL, 2003). The aging of Cuba has been rapid and intense. This success can be seen in Table 12.1 below:

Table 12.1   Demographic Portrait of Cuba (ONE, 2007)

Total population	11,239,043 residents
Population 60 years and older	1,779,994 (15.9%)
Life expectancy at birth	77 years
Life expectancy at 60 years	21.48 years
Life expectancy at 80 years	8.11 years

In spite of the material conditions of Cubans—subject to the U.S. blockade and the absence of a Socialist bloc since the fall of the Soviet Union—the state has maintained its principles of equity and equality and has continued to produce both qualitative and quantitative social policy changes, particularly in the areas of health, education, work, social security, and social justice (Saney, 2004). More than 60 percent of ongoing budgetary expenses go to health, education, social security, and social assistance (Oficina Nacional de Estadísticas [ONE], 2004; Rodríguez, 2000). The increase in life expectancy at birth is a reflection of a significant reduction in mortality over the last hundred years in Cuba and has resulted in a new challenge of caring for older adults, in a way that is consistent with the goals of the revolution. The appearance of specialized programs for certain groups has not happened by chance. It is the result of a well-planned health policy, limited economic resources, and an awareness of the need to guarantee care for the entire population, irrespective of ethnicity and social class, in a very humane way and with free access for all citizens.

Consequently, the health system has been planned to provide medical care focusing on specialized treatments. In order to accomplish this, medical and paramedical health personnel are trained to work in the different levels of primary, secondary, and tertiary care, so that there is continuity and interrelations between these three levels. The state has created different health programs according to the health needs of the population and the success of its health policy and planning is evidenced by health indicators that are comparable to countries at the highest level of development (Canadian International Development Agency [CIDA], 2007).

These programs have constituted an excellent way of bringing extended and secure attention to the populations in need, with the basic principle being primary health care. Primary health care occurs in the community, in direct contact with the target population, allowing for reliable firsthand knowledge. This assists in creating feasible solutions, not only for the individual in question and his or her family, but also in agreement with and through contact with the community in the expenditure of local or non-local resources. The growth in the number and proportion of older adults has motivated special attention from the state, in particular the Cuban Ministry of Public Health. Health-care practitioners find that older adults have more chronic diseases than younger people and, as a result, require more social and health services. While it is recognized that the majority of older adults are in good enough health that they will remain free of disability (National Institute on Aging, 2001), a significant proportion will become "frail" and require care or institutionalization, often for the rest of their lives. This is costly, as it calls for high-quality care that is multidimensional, integrated, and delivered where older adults live. Further, the gradual decline in physical and mental health conditions that accompanies the individual aging process, the resulting reduction in healthy and active life expectancy, and the reduction or complete cessation of labor-force participation, suggest that the growth in the oldest population will lead to an increased demand for health and social services (Vega et al., 2000).

With respect to demographic transitions such as these, a figure that is thought to be more important than the age in percentage is the dependency ratio or "burden of support" (Robertson, 1997), which is essentially the number of older people relative to younger people (Gee, 2002). Latin America is expected to have a dependency population increase from 7.3 percent in the year 2000 to 10.6 percent by the year 2050 (Harwood, Hirschfeld, & Sayer, 2004). There is strong criticism of the dependency ratio as an accurate measurement tool, however, as it arbitrarily assigns people into dependent and nondependent categories (Gee, 2000; Katz, 1990; Robertson, 1990; Vincent, 1996) and ignores the fact that any increase in older people and the accompanying costs will be offset by more people over age sixty-five choosing to remain in the workforce. Furthermore, the underlying assumption is that an increase in older people means an increase in people experiencing physiological decline, which is thought to equate aging with infirmity (Katz, 1990). Associating old age with dependency is no longer valid, however, as older people are better educated, in better health, and are staying in the workforce longer than ever before; dependency ratios do not account for older people doing unpaid work such as caregiving, grandparenting, or volunteering, or for potential migration trends (Gee, 2002; Wilson, 2002). A structured economic analysis of U.S. data discovered that the economic burden of an aging population will be no greater than that of raising the baby boomers of the 1960s (Knickman & Snell, 2002). Nonetheless, caring for older adults in the context of an aging society has been the focus of much debate and has resulted in numerous policy documents.

In Cuba, the first program for integrated care of the older adult was developed in 1974 and was later modified for inclusion in family doctor and nursing programs. In 1996, further revisions led to a new program with an integrated and multidisciplinary team focus based on international gerontological concepts. Once this program was in place, older adults could be incorporated into promotion and prevention activities, and this in turn led to an increase in the quality of assistance and community rehabilitation. The National Program for Integrated Care of the Older Adult, as it was called at the time, had three subprograms: community care, institutional care, and hospital care. The National Secretariat for the Older Adult and Social Assistance, created a unique program in which all levels and factors were addressed. This permitted a more integrated assessment and led to successes in terms of healthy aging, maintaining personal relationships, and participation of the family and community. Most of these areas were the responsibility of medicine and family nursing.

Medical Care for the Older Adult in Primary Care

The community care subprogram consists of the following programs or services for older adults: multidisciplinary gerontological care teams (EMAG); geriatric services; grandparents' circles; professors of older adults (under the auspices of the Cuban Workers Federation, the University of Havana, and the Cuban Teachers' Association); community and home-care services; social and domiciliary care; telephone help and advice services in some municipalities in the country; and sheltered housing.

The programs addressed care for the entire population of people age sixty years and older and broke this down into four areas: the search for chronic diseases and acute infections; noninfectious chronic diseases including arterial hypertension, diabetes mellitus, high cholesterol, obesity, and cognitive deterioration; achieving early cancer diagnosis; and guaranteeing gastro-intestinal care. Dementia, as a form of cognitive deterioration, falls within the detection of chronic diseases. In spite of the fact that few outstanding methods of preventing dementia exist to date, apart from reducing one's risk factors such as toxic habits and vascular disease, there is hope for the future.

As the relationship between cognitive deterioration, aging, and risk factors is well established, devising a strategy for the early detection of risk factors and cognitive deterioration is possible, particularly for Alzheimer's disease and other forms of dementia. This gives practitioners a reliable and valid method for trying to understand the illness and its diagnosis and acting upon related risk factors. In addition, it is important to consider the socioeconomic conditions in which these older adults and their families live, and to detect risk of falling in the home and in the community and the overall functional state of the older adult. These actions allow for planning with the family and the older adult, focusing on the possible progression of the illness and approaches for each phase, with a goal of maintaining persons living with dementia in their home, with their loved ones and their neighbors, in their community. A multidisciplinary team working in partnership with the community and in close contact with the family and the older adult with dementia carries out these activities.

Assessment of Older Adults with Cognitive Deterioration

The assessment that is undertaken in primary health care is guided by the principles of the Comprehensive Geriatric Assessment (VGI) protocol and is comprised of four parts: biomedical, psychological/cognitive, social, and functional. The purpose is to assess and manage cognitive deterioration in older adults through diagnosis and treatment, as well as to improve the quality of life of older people with dementia and their families. The most frequently used form is the one for Alzheimer's disease, which classifies AD in one of the following ways: antecedents of AD in the family (one or more cases among first-degree relatives), called familial Alzheimer's; no family antecedents, classified as sporadic Alzheimer's. To be considered early onset of either the familial or the sporadic form, the symptoms must have started prior to sixty-five years of age. In the overwhelming majority of cases, the first symptoms appear after sixty-five years of age, called late-onset Alzheimer's (Saido, 2003; Zarranz, 1997).

Among the nongenetic risk factors linked to AD are advanced age, family history of dementia in one or more first-degree relatives, female gender (mainly after eighty years), Down syndrome, cerebral trauma with loss of consciousness of more than one hour in duration, low educational level and intellectual quotient, diabetes mellitus, toxic habits, an early spontaneous or surgical menopause, and arterial hypertension (Diamond, 2006; García et al., 2002; Lindsay et al., 2002). At the present time, the most reliable markers of AD are neuropsychological: short-term memory loss verified by different tests and alterations in some executive functioning indicate cognitive changes that go beyond normal aging. The fourth edition of the *Diagnostic and Statistical Manual* (*DSM-IV*) (American Psychological Association, 1994) clearly sets out the diagnostic criteria for two subtypes of Alzheimer's dementia: early onset and late onset. This can be easily used in clinical practice by primary-health-care practitioners. It is important, once the preliminary diagnosis has been obtained, to approach the relatives and/or principal caregivers with a proposed care plan that will maintain function and slow the disease progression as much as possible for the older adult with dementia, for example, through the treatment and control of conditions that pose risks for vascular disease.

During the assessment of an older adult, the practitioner will often observe that social problems are a high priority and notice the ways in which these affect the health of the older adult; this is important for appropriate case management and to determine which factors to pay attention to and evaluate in establishing a diagnosis. Alzheimer's-type dementia should be viewed as a complex disease, not only in terms of diagnosis, but also in relation to psycho-econo-social considerations, such as the quality of life of the person with dementia and his or her family members. It is clear that this view of AD cannot be achieved if we do not know with accuracy the context surrounding those older adults whose cognitive function has been affected.

In Cuba, comprehensive assessment of each older adult showing signs of dementia is undertaken by EMAG, a multidisciplinary gerontological care group dedicated to integrated community care for older adults. The EMAG group offers support to the family-medicine team and foments other formal and informal community care directed at elevating the quality of life of older adults. It falls under the direction of the neighborhood polyclinic and forms a basic work group (GBT). As such, it does not supplant the activities carried out by the other members of the primary-care team; rather, EMAG organizes and leads the Program for Community Care of the Older Adult. Although their basic sphere of action is the community environment, EMAG also acts as a link from the polyclinic to the hospital and with social institutions. An EMAG team is composed of a doctor, nurse, psychologist, and social worker. The overall objective of an EMAG assessment is to respond to the needs and desires of the older adult and his or her family members. This group of professionals supplements the biopsychosocial care and rehabilitation offered by the GBT, in the hopes of avoiding institutionalization at all costs, favoring the acquisition of a better level of autonomy for the older adult, and proposing community solutions to problems.

The work of EMAG is always multidisciplinary and intersectoral and includes rehabilitation and treatment programs; physical exercises, physiotherapy, and occupational therapy; support for health prevention, promotion, and education programs; memory training for people with mild cognitive impairment or mild dementia and activities to maintain the functional capacity of people with dementia; and work related to the social-support programs of the Ministry of Work and Social Security, including interventions with families, together with the Basic Health Team. Working with families could involve family meetings, the provision of support to family members (self-help and mutual aid groups), or ensuring the participation of relatives.

EMAG is supported by the Popular Council, an entity that is integrated through representatives of different government sectors, such as the ministries of Work and Social Security and Culture; the National Institute of Sports Physical Education and Recreation (INDER); and the Commission on Prevention and Social Care. It is also supported by mass organizations such as Committees for the Defense of the Revolution (CDR), health brigades of the Cuban Federation of Women (FMC), and self-help and mutual aid groups. These groups participate in organizing and carrying out social and health initiatives designed to improve the quality of life of older adults.

Through VGI, older adults with dementia are classified as "frail older adults" and their needs ranked according to assigned risk: (1) evidence of minimal risk—older adult could benefit from health prevention and promotion; (2) stable chronic disease with risk factors that do not yet make one "needy"—early detection and use of primary and secondary health prevention and promotion; (3) chronic disease with obvious social needs that call for a caregiver—start of long-term care planning and biosocial attention to avoid functional deterioration, as well as caregiver education; (4) "frail elderly" with multiple biomedical, social, and functional problems with high risk of functional decline, hospital or institutional care, and death.

In the case of older adults who fall into groups three and four, the nurse and the social worker interview the family to determine the social environment (including social networks, social support, family relationships, and the workload of the potential caregiver); the environment in which the older adult became ill; the degree of support and assistance on which the family can count; and available community support services (how much from the community, from the state, from nongovernmental organizations, etc.). After completing this interview, they share this information with the rest of the EMAG team and complete the patient record using the Geronte graphic record, which gives a panoramic view of any deficiencies in the older adult's functioning. They then develop an individual plan for each older adult, listing the care needed and resources available and look for the items needed to achieve a solution. As many organizations as possible are involved to support this intervention, which may include gero-activities of the CDRs, the FMC, and the community, in an effort to create solutions that meet the needs of the older adult.

Community Care for Older Adults

Such ongoing attention in the community reduces the cost of prolonged medical care, helps to avoid crises, and ensures the needs of older adults will be discovered and addressed. However, the attention received by older adults as a special group is controversial in Cuba, with some people feeling that older adults should receive services according to this format and others arguing that their needs should be attended along with services designed for the general population.

Case Study—Mary

EMAG received a referral from the medical consultation in the health area (Medical Clinic of Primary Health Care, in Cuba "Clinic of the Doctor of the Family") for a sixty-seven-year-old Afro-Cuban woman—an active smoker with pathological antecedents including hypertension, high cholesterol, and type 2 diabetes mellitus. The nurse in the basic work group referred this woman, Mary, to the medical clinic after she had conducted a home visit (for patients with chronic diseases), and

Mary's relative (the son with whom she lives) told the nurse that Mary had changed over the past two months. Mary was not able to make purchases in the market because she lost money or she forgot what she had meant to buy. This situation caused irritability, and on occasion she had accused her son of "stealing her belongings," because she couldn't find them. In addition, the son noted that a few days previously when Mary was in the kitchen, she had forgotten to turn off the burner, and hence the food she was preparing burned. Some adjacent neighbors found her crying and immediately located her son at his workplace. The son was very alarmed because they lived alone, his mother was getting worse all the time, and he needed to work. They had no other relatives or close friends to help them.

The EMAG consultation was initiated and Mary was evaluated multi-dimensionally and comprehensively by each of the team members, through a geriatric assessment that includes biomedical, psychological, social, and functional components.

BIOMEDICAL ASSESSMENT

Through the physical exam and health questionnaire, the doctor determined that Mary had blood chemistry within a normal range, and the simple tomography of the skull showed cortical diffuse atrophy. The rest of the tests yielded normal results.

PSYCHOLOGICAL ASSESSMENT

When the psychologist went deeper into the clinical history through interviewing her relative (because Mary didn't recall the following), they determined that the cognitive deterioration dated no more than three years. The son had been working all day and arriving home tired, so he had been missing certain details, which now became clearer. For example, his mother frequently stopped paying the electricity bill, or left the door open, and she even forgot important festival dates. She did not remember giving messages and showed evidence of perseveration on certain topics. She frequently claimed that "they" took her things, such as her money and her clothes.

Recently, the son had had to take on making purchases for the household because Mary was forgetting what she should buy or how much she should pay. She always repeated conversations as if they were new, with a tendency to remember the past and to speak of family or friends who had died as if they were still alive. On occasion, without apparent reason, she had been found crying and disinterested in her personal care; plus, she seemed irritable and almost aggressive (verbally and nonverbally). Mary described episodes of complex illusions and confusion in identification and thought strange people were living in the house.

When the Mini Mental examination (MMSE) was administered, the psychologist took into account that Mary had completed high school–level schooling and had no sensory limitations. She had a good level of attention, but had a lot of difficulty with orientation to space and time, as well as with memory and language and was incapable of reproducing a polygon. She scored thirteen points out of a possible thirty on the MMSE. She scored a 2 on the Clinical Dementia Rating (CDR) scale. Applying the *DSM-IV* criteria led to the conclusion that Mary could be classified as having a probable Dementing Syndrome.

SOCIAL ASSESSMENT

Through assessment by the team social worker, we learned that this was a nuclear family, mother and son. The father had died three years previously, as a consequence of cerebrovascular disease and, since then, Mary had appeared sad on occasion, yet was active and took care of the home in an efficient way.

The son had university-level education, worked as an electrical engineer for a business, and his wage along with the pension from Mary's husband covered their basic needs. However, the son's work occupied him for a great part of the day, and thus Mary was spending time on her own. Some neighbors were helping her with the market and sometimes with heating food that the son left for her. Lately, something had been making Mary irritable though, so sometimes she wouldn't let the neighbors into the house. Recently, she had left the house, and they had found her nearby; she did not know how to return home.

The social worker used the Caregiver's Scale and found areas in which the son was fed up with the situation. In the home, there appeared to be architectural barriers that posed "risks because they produce falls"; for example, the house only had one bedroom, with big furniture in it, which was difficult for Mary to pass through. There was inadequate nighttime illumination because the bathroom was far from the bedroom and there was no nightlight to help Mary find her way should the need arise.

FUNCTIONAL ASSESSMENT

Mary demonstrated total dependence for all instrumental activities of daily living, on the basis of Lawton's scale, which is why her contact with the surrounding area was very limited. As for the basic activities of daily living (Katz's Index), the nurse registered that Mary was independent for eating and controlling her sphincter, but not for the rest of the activities.

EMAG concluded that in this case the following diagnoses converged:

- Diagnostic Group: III. Probable Dementing Syndrome: moderate stage (the cortical profile suggested Alzheimer's disease but a neuropsychological assessment was requested)

- Limited support network

- Burned-out caregiver

- High risk of falling: architectural barriers

In this case, the team's report led to Mary being assigned a caregiver (a neighbor who did not work) to help during the day with Mary's care while her son was working. The team provided the son with comprehensive information on his mother's disease, including the expected progression, key characteristics, and care required at each stage of the illness, through to the final stages. The team recommended that the son attend Caregivers School, depending on his free time. In this activity, relatives sharing a similar situation meet together and are guided by trained personnel who help them with information on the care of people with dementia. Finally, the team sent a summary for Mary's clinical history in primary care, so that they could follow up with her.

This case demonstrated how EMAG works to comprehensively assess an older adult showing signs of cognitive deterioration in a holistic and interdisciplinary fashion and then develops a care plan that will enable the older adult with dementia to remain in her home community with necessary supports. In this case, a neighbor was designated as Mary's caregiver so that her son could continue working and she could remain in her home. This chapter ends with brief reflections from each of the authors.

Reflections of a Canadian Dementia Researcher

There has been much talk in the dementia field of the need to consider people with dementia as unique beings who reside in diverse sociocultural contexts. The Cuban approach to dementia care accomplishes this, as shown through the above descriptions of primary health care, Community Care for the Older Adult, and EMAG, plus the case study of an older adult showing signs of cognitive deterioration. Cuban dementia care clearly foregrounds context and supports the idea of dementia-friendly communities, not through an intentional approach such as that promoted in the global North (Alzheimer Scotland Action on Dementia, 2001; Marshall, 1999), but rather as a natural consequence of viewing all persons as human beings who are part of a shared struggle for humanity, equity, and social justice, and who are members of communities, not only individuals.

Reflections of a Cuban Doctor

The difficulties under which Cuba struggles are well known; however, another reality is that the graduates of Cuban medical schools enjoy prestige throughout the world. One has to wonder how it is possible that, faced with so many economic difficulties, we stay on our feet, with excellent health in our health-care system—a small and blockaded country.

Those of us who have the privilege of being able to practice medicine in Cuba don't see behind our patients a figure, a price, a gain, or an improvement in our status in life; we see the human being and his or her family in a complete context, very near to our own lives and our daily problems, because we are from Cuba and we live in Cuba.

Our medicine is human, disinterested and scientific, and those who know us know that we are people who lend a hand: we embrace the wounded and aching ones, we suffer for those who suffer, and we are capable of looking for alternatives amongst all the options, with few resources, without ever losing the perspective of human beings who want to live more, but with quality of life.

References

10/66 Dementia Research Group. (2000). Dementia in developing countries: A consensus statement from the 10/66 Dementia Research Group. *International Journal of Geriatric Psychiatry, 15*, 14–20.

10/66 Dementia Research Group. (2004). Care arrangements for people with dementia in developing countries. *International Journal of Geriatric Psychiatry, 19*, 170–177.

Albala, C., Lebrão, M. L., León Díaz, E. M., Ham-Chande, R., Hennis, A. J., Palloni, A., et al. (2005). Encuesta salud, bienestar y envejecimiento (SABE): Metodología de la encuestra y perfil de la población estudiada. *Rev Panam Salud Publica/Pan Am J Public Health, 17*(5/6), 307–322.

Alzheimer Scotland Action on Dementia. (2001). *Creating dementia-friendly communities*. Edinburgh, Scotland: Alzheimer Scotland Action on Dementia.

American Psychological Association. (1994). *Diagnostic and statistical manual of mental disorders* (4th ed.). Washington, DC: American Psychological Association.

Anuario Estadístico. (2006). La Habana, CU: ONE-MINSAP.

Baggio, G., Donazzan, S., Monti, D., Mari, D., Martini, S., Gabelli, C., et al. (1998). Lipoprotein(a) and lipoprotein profile in healthy centenarians: A reappraisal of vascular risk factors. *FASEB J, 12*(6), 433–437.

Bertera, E. (2003). Social services for the aged in Cuba [electronic version]. *International Social Work, 46*(3), 313–321.

Brink, S. (1997). The graying of our communities worldwide [electronic version]. *Ageing International, Winter/Spring,* 13–31.

Canadian Institutes of Health Research (CIHR). (2007). *The future is aging: The CIHR Institute of Aging strategic plan 2007–2012.* Retrieved June 18, 2007, from http://www.cihr-irsc.gc.ca/cgi-bin/print-imprimer.pl

Canadian International Development Agency (CIDA). (2007). *Cuba: Facts at a glance.* Retrieved February 9, 2008, from http://www.acdicida.gc.ca/CIDAWEB/acdicida.nsf/En/NIC223122134-ND2

Canadian Study of Health and Aging (CSHA) Working Group. (1994). Canadian study of health and aging: Study methods and prevalence of dementia. *Canadian Medical Association Journal, 150*(60), 899–913.

Carrasco, M. M., & Blas, S. J. (2004). Mild cognitive impairment: A necessary entity? *INTERSIQUIS,* 15–23.

Carrasco, M. R. (2001). Trabajo de investigación del Grupo Alzheimer del Cerro. Pesquisaje de Deterioro Cognitivo en adultos mayores del Policlínico Cerro. Ciudad de la Habana.

CEPAL. (2003). *Conferencia Regional intergubernamental sobre envejecimiento: Una estrategia regional de implementación para América Latina y el Caribe del Plan de Acción Internacional de Madrid obre el envejecimiento.* Documento de Referencia DDR/1. Preparado por: División de Población de la CEPAL/Centro Latinoamericano y Caribeño de Demografía (CELADE)/Grupo de trabajo interinstitucional sobre el envejecimiento: La Organización Panamericana de la Salud (OPS)/el Fondo de Población de las Naciones Unidas (UNFPA), la Organización Internacional del Trabajo (OIT), el Banco Interamericano de Desarrollo (BID), el Banco Mundial y el Programa sobre el Envejecimiento de las Naciones Unidas. Santiago de Chile, 19–21 de noviembre.

CEPDE. (2005). *Cuba 10 años después de la Conferencia Internacional sobre la Población y el Desarrollo.* La Habana, 6–7.

De la Torre, J., & Hachinski, V. (Eds.). (2002). Alzheimer´s disease as a vascular disorder: Nosological evidence. *Stroke, 58,* 1587–1588.

Diamond, J. (2006). *A report on Alzheimer disease and current research.* (Revised ed.). Toronto, Canada: Alzheimer Society of Canada.

Ebrahim, S. (2002). Ageing, health and society. *International Journal of Epidemiology, 31,* 715–718.

Ferri, C. P., Prince, M., Brayne, C., Brodaty, H., Fratiglioni, L., Ganguli, M., et al. (2005). Global prevalence of dementia: A Delphi consensus study. *Lancet, 366,* 2112–2117.

Fillit, H., & O'Concell, A. (2002). *Drug discovery and development for Alzheimer's Disease.* New York: Springer Publishing Company.

Florez-Tascón Sixto, F. J., Florez-Tascón, F. J., Carreras, D. S., Vega, S. Q., Valderrama, M. L., & Collado, M. A. (2003). Alzheimer´s disease clinic in 2003. *Geriatrika, 19*(Supl. 1), 27–36.

García, F. G., Rodríguez, J., & Jiménez, G. (2002). Evaluación neuropsicológica en el anciano. En documentos técnicos de la Sociedad Española de Geriatría y Gerontología: Demencias. *Rev Esp Geriatr Gerontol, 37*(Supl. 4), 10–25.

Gee, E. (2000). Population and politics: Voodoo demography, population aging and social policy. In E. Gee & G. Gutman (Eds.), *The overselling of population*

aging: Apocalyptic demography, intergenerational challenges and social policy (pp. 5–25). Don Mills, Canada: Oxford University Press.

Gee, E. (2002). Misconceptions and misapprehensions about population ageing. *International Journal of Epidemiology, 31,* 750–753.

Gondor, A., & Negrin, E. (1998). *Aging in Cuba: Realities and changes.* Retrieved March 22, 2005, from http://www.globalaging.org/elderrights/world/cuba .htm

Graff-Radford, N. R., Crook, J. E., Lucas, J., Boeve, B. F., Knopman, D. S., Ivnick, R. J., et al. (2007). Association of low plasma $A\beta42/A\beta40$ ratios with increased imminent risk for mild cognitive impairment and Alzheimer's disease. *Archives of Neurology, 64,* 354–362.

Harwood, R., Hirschfeld, M., & Sayer, A. (2004). Current and future worldwide prevalence of dependency ratios [electronic version]. *Bulletin of the World Health Organization, 82*(4), 251–258.

Hernández Pérez Y. (1999). *Prevalencia y factores de riesgo de discapacidad en ancianos. Municipio Puerto Padre y Las Tunas. [Trabajo para optar por el título de Especialista de Primer Grado en Bioestadística].* La Habana, Cuba: Facultad de Salud Pública.

Herrera-Valdés, R., & Almaguer-López, M. (2005). Strategies for national health care systems and centres in the emerging world: Central America and the Caribbean—the case of Cuba. *Kidney International, 68*(S98), S66–S68.

Kane, L., Ouslander, R., & Abrass, I. B. (2000). *Geriatría Clínica* [translated from the 4th English edition of *Essential Clinical Geriatrics*]. Interamericana Editores, S.A. de C.V., México: McGraw-Hill.

Katz, S. (1990). Alarmist demography: Power, knowledge and the elderly population. *Journal of Aging Studies, 6*(3), 203–225.

Knickman, J., & Snell, E. (2002). The 2030 problem: Caring for aging baby boomers [electronic version]. *Health Services Research, 37*(4), 849–884.

Lindsay, J., Laurin, D., Verreault, R., Hébert, R., Helliwell, B., Hill, G. B., McDowell, I. (2002). Risk factors for Alzheimer's disease: A prospective analysis from the Canadian Study of Health and Aging. *Am J Epidemiol, 156*(5), 445–453.

Llibre Rodríguez, J. J., & Hernández, M. G. (2002). Actualización de la enfermedad de Alzheimer. *Rev Cub Med Gen Integral, 4,* 12–14.

Lussier, I., Malenfant, D., Peretz, I., & Beleville, S. (2001). Caractérisation des troubles de la mémoire dans la démence de type Alzheimer. In M. Dans Habib, Y. Joanette, & M. Puel (Eds.), *Démences et syndromes démentiels: Approche neuropsychologique.* Paris: Masson.

Makoto Higuchi, F. H. (2005). MRI detection of amyloid plaques in vivo. *Nat Neurosci,* advance online publication, 13 March.

Marshall, M. (1999). What do service planners and policy-makers need from research? *International Journal of Geriatric Psychiatry, 14,* 86–96.

Martínez Lage, P., Hachinski, V., Martínez Lage, J. M. (2001). Senilidad cerebral evitable: La importancia de eludir las enfermedades cerebrovasculares demenciantes. In *Envejecimiento cerebral y ynfermedad* (pp. 351–373). Madrid, Spain: Tricastela.

Monti D., Salvioli, S., Capri, M., Malorni, W., Straface, E., Cossarizza, A., et al. (2000). Inherited variability of the mitochondrial genome and successful aging in humans. *Ann N Y Acad Sci, 908,* 208–218.

National Institute on Aging. (2001, May 7). Dramatic decline in disability continues for older Americans. Retrieved March 15, 2009, from http://www.nia.nih .gov/NewsAndEvents/PressReleases/PR20010507Dramatic.htm

National Institute on Aging. (2007). 2007 progress report on Alzheimer's Disease. Discovery and hope. Retrieved March 15, 2009, from http://www.nia.nih.gov

National Institute on Aging. (2008, September). Alzheimer's disease: Unraveling the mystery. Retrieved March 15, 2009, from http://www.nia.nih.gov

Oficina Nacional de Estadísticas (ONE). (enero, 2004). *Panorama Económico y Social de Cuba, 2003.*

Oficina National de Estadísticas (ONE). (2007). *Anuario estadístico de Cuba 2006.* Retrieved March 28, 2008, from http://www.one.cu/aec2006.htm

Ognibene, A., Petruzzi, E., Troiano, L., Pini, G., Franceschi, C., Monti, D., et al. (1999).Testosterone, gonadotropins, prolactin and sex hormone-binding globulin in healthy centenarians. *J Endocrinol Invest, 22*(Suppl. 10), 64–65.

Parkin, A. L. (2001). *Memory: Phenomena, experiment and theory.* Oxford, England: Blackwell.

Pliacentini, M., Baggio, G., Barbi, C., Valensin, S., Bonafe, M., & Franceschi, C. (2000). Decreased susceptibility to oxidative stress-induced apoptosis of peripheral blood mononuclear cells from healthy elderly and centenarians. *Mech Ageing Dev, 121*(1–3), 239–250.

Prince, M., Acosta, D., Chui, H., Scazufca, M., & Varghese, M. (2003). Dementia diagnosis in developing countries: A cross-cultural validation study. *Lancet, 361,* 909–917.

Robertson, A. (1990). The politics of Alzheimer's disease: A case study of apocalyptic demography. *International Journal of Health Services, 20*(3), 429–442.

Robertson, A. (1997). Beyond apocalyptic demography: Towards a moral economy of interdependence. *Ageing & Society, 17,* 425–446.

Robine, J. M., & Vaupel, J. W. (2001). Supercentenarians: Slower ageing individuals or senile elderly? *Experimental Gerontology, 36*(9), 15–30.

Rodríguez, J. L. (2000). *Cuba: El camino de la recuperación económica y el informe sobre los resultados económicos de 1999 y el plan económico para el año 2000.*

Saido, T. C. (2003). Overview of AB metabolism: From Alzheimer. In T. C. Saido (Ed.), *AB metabolism and Alzheimer's Disease* (ch. 2). Austin, Texas: Landes Bioscience. Retrieved March 11, 2009, from http://www.landesbioscience.com/ curie/chapter/896

Sánchez, Y. (2006, February 17). *Resultados de la investigáción sobre la dementia en Cuba: Presentáción a los participantes.* Centro Communitario de la Salud Mental, Playa. Havana, Cuba.

Saney, I. (2004). *Cuba: A revolution in motion.* Halifax, NS: Fernwood Publishing.

Shaji, K. S., Smitha, K., Praveen Lal, K., & Prince, M. J. (2003). Caregivers of people with Alzheimer's disease: A qualitative study from the Indian 10/66 dementia research network. *International Journal of Geriatric Psychiatry, 18,* 1–6.

Strug, D. (2004). An exploratory study of social work with older persons in Cuba: Implications for social work in the U.S. [electronic version]. *Journal of Gerontological Social Work, 43*(2/3), 25–40.

Vega, E. G., Menéndez, J. J., Diéguez, R. D., Martínez, L. A., Baly, M. B., Arencibia, H. P., et al. (2000). Dirección Nacional de Adulto Mayor y Asistencia Social, Cuba.

Vincent, J. (1996). Who's afraid of an ageing population? Nationalism, the free market and the construction of old age as an issue. *Critical Social Policy, 47*(16), 3–26.

Wilson, G. (2002). Globalisation and older people: Effects of markets and migration. *Ageing & Society, 22*, 647–663.

Wilson, R. S., Mendes, C. F., Barnes, L. L., Schneider, J. A., Evans, D. A., & Bennett, D. A. (2002). Participation in cognitively stimulating activities and risk of incidence of Alzheimer's disease. *JAMA, 287*, 742–747.

Zarranz, J. J. (1997). Alteraciones morfológicas y neuroquímicas en el envejecimiento cerebral normal. *Rev Neurol, 25*(Supl. 1), S9–S13.

CHAPTER THIRTEEN

Social Work with the Frail Elderly in Cuba: The Importance of Social Capital

David L. Strug

This chapter explores the importance of social capital in social work with the frail elderly in Cuba. It describes how Cuban social workers access social relationships, ties and networks among neighbors, community organizations, and health professionals—social capital—to help the frail elderly get health care and social assistance. It shows that social work in Cuba is integrated into the public-health system of the community, which facilitates social workers' access to sources of social capital. Two case examples illustrate this point.

The primary questions this chapter addresses are the following: (1) How is social work integrated into the health-care system of the community? (2) How does this integration allow social workers access to social capital to help the frail elderly? and, (3) Can social workers in the United States benefit by learning how their Cuban counterparts access sources of social capital to help frail older adults?

Frail, or fragile, older adults include elderly persons with limited physical mobility and cognitive capacity, or who lack family support or economic resources. These limitations interfere with their ability to carry out daily activities and, in some instances, to live independently (Alonso Galbán, Sansó Soberats, Díaz-Canel Navarro, Carrasco García, & Oliva, 2007). Social workers in Cuba by enhancing social capital play an important role in helping fragile older adults remain in the community.

Social capital is a concept that is not widely known in the U.S. social work community (Midgeley & Livermore, 1998). Social capital represents a feature of community social organization and is a resource that can facilitate collective action in the neighborhood. It is associated with civic participation in voluntary associations, with norms of mutual aid, and with reciprocity (Lochner, Kawachi, & Kennedy, 1999). Social capital is connected with the amount of effort that a network of concerned individuals in a community makes on behalf of a particular individual or group (Carnoy, 2007). Investigators have demonstrated a robust relationship between social capital and the health of community members (Folland, 2007). Trusting and socially active individuals, as opposed to individuals with lower levels of trust and civic participation, more often report good or very good health in countries with high levels of social capital (Poortinga, 2006).

Social workers, health professionals, and civic associations in Cuba work together to address health and social problems related to aging. Social workers concerned with the elderly in the United States can benefit from examining how Cuban social workers access sources of social capital to help older adults, even though the two countries have different economic, political, and social systems.

Cuba's Aging Population

There is little information in the United States, or in the Cuban social work literature, about Cuba's growing elderly population (Bertera, 2003; Goicoechea-Balbona & Conill-Mendoza, 2000; Strug, 2004). This is surprising, given the significance that a rapidly aging population has for Cuban social policy makers and for the social work profession on the island. Cuba has one of the oldest populations in Latin America, and it is growing rapidly (Rodríguez, Castellón, & Puga Gonzalez, 2004). More than 16 percent of Cuba's population (18% of Havana's) is currently age sixty and older (Arreola, 2008), and by 2025 one in four Cubans will be over sixty (Giraldo, 2007). Cuba has many innovative approaches for addressing the growth of the older population and their needs (Bertera, 2003) and has extensive gerontology and geriatrics programs, which employ many social workers.

A major survey of persons age sixty and older conducted in 2000 indicated that approximately half of Cuba's older population (51%) lived with other people and 22 percent lived alone or with a spouse (Centro Iberoamericano de la Tercera Edad, 2005). More than 90 percent received outside help in the form of financial assistance, social services, or some other type of aid. More than two-thirds of older Cubans (70%) have at least one chronic illness, with arthritis, arterial hypertension, heart disease, cognitive deterioration, and cancer more common in those age seventy-five and older (Centro Iberoamericano de la Tercera Edad, 2005). About half of all the medical services sought in 2000 were with family doctors. Cubans live about as long as their U.S. counterparts (77.6 years for Cubans versus 77.7 for the Americans), despite the fact that Cuba is a poor, nonindustrialized country. This impressive life expectancy is related to the fact that Cuba has an outstanding health-care system (MEDICC, 2007).

Population aging has occurred during a time of great economic adversity in Cuba due to the collapse of the Soviet Union, on which the island was economically dependent, in 1990. The U.S. trade embargo has also economically harmed Cuba. These factors affect the elderly in particular. Economic problems limit the size of pensions the government can pay retired persons. Many elderly people must depend on family members to assist in the purchase of food and clothing, because pensions and social assistance for the elderly are typically not sufficient to cover the cost of these items. Older Cubans who live alone have an especially difficult time surviving economically. The elderly are affected by a shortage of medical supplies resulting from the U.S. trade embargo. At the same time, the government has sent more than thirty thousand Cuban doctors abroad to work on international humanitarian medical missions, mostly to Venezuela (MEDICC, 2009). Older Cubans are especially affected by the export of these doctors, because the elderly have a greater need for medical attention than do younger persons.

The government introduced a National Plan of Assistance to Older Adults in 2003 (CEPAL, 2004), increased social security payments to the elderly, added a number of interventions to support the needs of frail older adults in their homes, and began a Substitute Family Program that attempts to place older adults no longer able to live alone with a foster family in the neighborhood (Águila & Jubán, 2002). The Substitute Family Program is an example of the government's promotion of a communal ethos, or a tradition of popular participation of community residents and of locally elected representatives in neighborhood social-action programs.

The community became the central locus for new social development and prevention efforts and for delivering services to the elderly and other vulnerable groups in the mid nineties (Uriarte, 2002). International organizations, local authorities, so-called mass organizations, and neighborhood residents became involved in construction, environmental protection, and other types of community-development projects (Dilla, 1999). Mass organizations, such as the Federation of Cuban Women (FMC), are entities created after the Cuban Revolution that are entrusted with a variety of public health, educational, and security functions at different levels of Cuban society, from the neighborhood to the national level (Díaz-Briquets, 2002). Mass organizations participate in many aspects of the Cuban health-care system, and social workers regularly interact with these entities in their work with the elderly. The central government has delegated to regional local authorities and to mass organizations the responsibility of identifying vulnerable populations including the frail elderly, with special service needs and determining ways of meeting those needs.

Study Methods and Limitations

Information for this chapter comes primarily from twenty-nine qualitative, open-ended interviews that the author conducted in two Havana neighborhoods in the summer of 2005 and 2006. These interviews were conducted with ten social workers, eight health professionals, five representatives of mass organizations, and six elderly community members. Information also comes from a review of the literature on social work and on the Cuban health-care system.

Interview questions for social workers concerned their role in the health system, their work with older persons both in municipal clinics and in the community, and their interaction with mass organizations. Health professionals other than social workers were asked about their work with social workers, with frail community members, and with mass organizations. Representatives of mass organizations were asked about their work with community members, their interaction with social workers, and their connection with the health-care system. Questions for frail older adults and other community members concerned their interaction with neighbors, with social workers, and with health professionals in the municipal clinic and in the community.

The interviews were tape-recorded and the audiotapes were transcribed. The author conducted an iterative content analysis, studied the text methodically, and read and reviewed the transcribed material to identify common themes (e.g., accessing social relationships, decision making). Common thematic motifs were identified and transcript sections were singled out for comparison. This method is commonly used by investigators in qualitative research for the analysis of open-ended data (Creswell, 1994). The study results from this data analysis and from a review of the literature on social work and the Cuban health-care system are presented below.

This is an exploratory study, the sample size is small, and interviews took place in only two Havana neighborhoods. Also, the research was conducted over a comparatively short time interval. Therefore, study findings pose a problem for generalizing.

The Integration of Social Work into the Cuban Health-Care System

It is necessary to describe the integrated, multisectorial nature of the Cuban health system in order to explain how social work is integrated into that system. The Cuban health system is a decentralized one and is vertically integrated at the national, provincial, municipal, and neighborhood levels (Dresang, Brebrick, Murray, Shallue, & Sullivan-Vedder, 2005). The vertical integration of this three-tier health system allows a community-based approach to fit with secondary and tertiary levels of care (Pérez-Ávila, 2001). The Ministry of Public Health (MINSAP) coordinates all levels of health care at the national level. Hospital-based care represents one tier of the system and is located primarily at the provincial level. Polyclinics represent a second tier and are organized at the municipal level. A polyclinic is a municipal health-care center that offers many health and social services for nearby community members (Waller, 2002). Medical teams in the polyclinic operate according to a paradigm known as "medicine in the community," which treats patients as biopsychosocial beings in their respective, unique environments (Feinsilver, 1993). Polyclinics now provide many of the services and medical equipment previously available only at hospitals in an effort to increase availability of services to community members. Each municipality has one or more polyclinic, depending on the size of the municipality, and each polyclinic is divided into health sectors that serve multiple communities.

Family-medicine consultation centers are located at the community level and represent the third tier of Cuba's three-tiered health system. Primary care provided by a family doctor/nurse team represents a major element of the health-care system at the neighborhood level. Family doctor/nurse teams provide personalized primary health care from anywhere between 125 and 165 families at the block level. A family-practice office staffed by a doctor/nurse team (*consultorio*) addresses the majority of the health problems in the community and emphasizes health promotion. Doctor/nurse teams perform regular home visits, even visiting those in good health, thereby offering personalized attention to the individuals and families at greatest risk and facilitating preventive measures (Oficina Nacional de Estadísticas, 1998–1999). Family doctors also maintain close ties with the polyclinic, including with the social worker at the clinic.

The Cuban health-care system is also intersectorial and promotes health initiatives through coordination with local decision-making bodies, people's councils (PCs), and through the promotion of community participation in a variety of ways. PCs are an important link in Cuba's three-tiered health system. They function at a level that is between the municipality and the neighborhood in order to bridge decision making between the local community and the wider municipal level. A PC is comprised of community delegates and representatives of grassroots organizations, state enterprises, and administrative entities. It is a vehicle of decision making about meeting the economic, health, and social needs of community members under its jurisdiction (Roman, 2003) and therefore is an important source of social capital. PCs coordinate, control, and monitor the delivery of health care and other services that originate at the national level, and promote community participation in health care to assist the neighborhood in solving its health problems.

Social workers are integrated into interdisciplinary health-care teams within each level of Cuba's three-tier health system. They work with doctors, nurses, public-health officials in municipal hospitals, and in public-health offices throughout Cuba.

Health Social Work with the Elderly

Every Cuban polyclinic has an interdisciplinary gerontology team (EMAG, or *Equipo Multidisciplinario de Atención Gerontológica*), which is made up of a geriatric social worker, a specialist in comprehensive general medicine, a nurse, and a psychologist (Program of Attention to Older Persons, 2000). The social worker sees at-risk older adults for part of the day in the polyclinic and spends the rest of the time in the community working with older persons, with the doctor/nurse team, and with community representatives. The time that the social worker spends in the community and the interaction that the social worker has with community members distinguishes this worker's role from that of the other gerontology team members.

The social worker is the EMAG team member who is most familiar with the family environment of the older person. The social worker's knowledge of the social context in which the older person lives is critical to the team's overall health and psychosocial assessment. The social worker also assesses whether the older person is capable of remaining at home or must be placed in a day hospital, a nursing home, or an older person's daycare center, known as "a Grandparent's House" (*Casa de Abuelo*). A Grandparent's House is a day program for older persons, and such programs are located in municipalities throughout Cuba. The social worker also encourages the elderly to participate in activities established specifically for older adults, including grandparent's circles (*Círculos de Abuelos*) and orientation and recreation groups, or GORs (*Grupos de Orientación y Recreación*). Grandparent's circles offer physical activities, while the GORs offer field trips, arts and crafts, literary and acting workshops, movie debates, and health education and prevention activities (Giraldo, 2007).

Social Work, Mass Organizations, and Social Capital

Social workers participate in collaborative, community-based projects, whose goals are to improve the health and overall well-being of members of the community (Martínez Canals & García Brigos, 2001). Social workers are regular participants in people's council meetings, where they advocate for community members with special health-care and social-assistance needs or other problems. Social workers also participate in meetings of mass organizations, such as the Cuban Federation of Women (FMC) and the Committees for the Defense of the Revolution (CDR). They work with the FMC on major public-health initiatives such as vaccination campaigns (Coyula & Hamburg, 2007) and campaigns to eliminate dengue fever (Uriarte, 2002).

Two cases are presented below to show how social workers' integration into the health system facilitates their access to social capital and how this integration assists them in their work with frail older adults.

BARBARA'S NEED FOR FAMILY SUPPORT

Águila and Jubán (2002) described the involvement of an "empirical social worker" in a Havana neighborhood who became concerned about her eighty-seven-year-old neighbor, Barbara. An empirical social worker (*trabajador social empírico*) is a community member and a member of the Cuban Federation of Women who carries out an important social work role in the neighborhood, often with the assistance of the polyclinic social worker. The empirical social worker has no formal training in social work, but is a "social work volunteer" of the FMC. He or she receives an orientation in social work by this mass organization that allows the empirical social worker to be sensitive to the support-service needs of at-risk groups, including the frail elderly.

Barbara was suffering from deteriorating health conditions and had become increasingly dependent upon neighbors to assist her with activities of daily living. The older woman's neighbors felt overburdened by her requests for help and spoke with the empirical social worker about this matter. The empirical social worker contacted the social worker of the gerontology team at the nearby polyclinic for assistance. The gerontology team social worker discussed this case with her EMAG team members and with Barbara's family doctor in the community where Barbara lived. The worker then visited the elderly woman in her home along with the empirical social worker, and together they assessed Barbara's living situation. The social worker learned that Barbara was widowed, was receiving an inadequate pension, was living alone in a two-room, dilapidated apartment, and had no family members in the community to care for her. The polyclinic social worker together in consultation with the family doctor concluded that Barbara could no longer live alone because of her many physical ailments and because she needed more help than a part-time domestic aide could provide.

The polyclinic and the empirical social worker considered the possibility of finding a nursing home for Barbara. The waiting list for nursing home admission was a long one, however, and the workers preferred to find a way for the woman to remain in her community, near friends and neighbors. The social workers then made the decision to bring this case to a meeting of the people's council, made up of key individuals including the doctor and nurse from Barbara's community, a social worker from the municipal health department, the president of the people's council, and leaders of mass organizations, which included the Committee for the Defense of the Revolution (CDR). After a long discussion of Barbara's situation, the people's council recommended that the polyclinic and empirical social workers take Barbara's case before the Commission for the Prevention of Social Problems in Barbara's community for a final decision to be made at the local level. This commission is directed by the community delegate, or representative elected by community members, and is comprised of representatives of mass organizations and of other local officials of the community. It meets regularly to address social problems that concern the welfare of people in the neighborhood.

A special meeting of the Commission for the Prevention of Social Problems was convened, and it was attended by the social worker who informed the commission members of Barbara's deteriorated condition and need for support. The commission decided that the social workers should look for a substitute family in the community with whom the elderly woman might be able to live under the government's Substitute Family Program (Águila & Jubán, 2002). The commission's decision was authoritative because of its makeup, which included the most important community-level decision makers, and because the regional level people's council had charged the commission with the task of making a final decision about Barbara's situation.

The polyclinic and the empirical social workers were in agreement with this decision and were eventually able to identify an appropriate family willing to invite the eighty-seven-year-old woman to live in their home on a trial basis. Barbara accepted the family's offer, and the social workers arranged with the municipal office of the Ministry of Labor and Social Assistance for the substitute family to receive a small stipend to help defray expenses related to Barbara's living with them. The social workers monitored the process of adaptation of Barbara and the substitute family and arranged for Barbara to get the medical attention she needed with the family doctor in the community and at the polyclinic.

The social workers continued to monitor the situation until the elderly woman's death (O. G. Jubán, personal communication, November 25, 2003).

MARGARITA'S NEED FOR FINANCIAL AND MEDICAL ASSISTANCE

The case of Margarita illustrates how the polyclinic social worker and the community primary-care physician work closely to help the frail elderly receive financial and medical assistance. Margarita was an eighty-one-year-old widow who had lived with her brother, Jaime, for many years, until his death from a heart attack. Margarita now had to live alone, suffered from multiple sclerosis, and was wheelchair bound. She had to be carried out of the house by neighbors when she went outside, because the entrance to her house was connected to the street below by a series of steep steps. The lack of building materials in the community made it impossible for neighbors to construct a ramp, which would have facilitated her leaving her house by wheelchair.

Margarita's need for domestic and for financial assistance had increased dramatically since Jaime's death. Her deceased husband's social security pension was insufficient to cover all of her expenses, which her brother had helped to pay. Her family doctor, who lived across the street from Margarita, had been concerned about how Margarita would survive on her own since her brother died. The doctor had supplied her with some of his own food, because she did not have enough money to pay for all the food she needed. He contacted the polyclinic social worker, with whom the doctor had worked for many years, and together they sought domestic help for Margarita through the Social Assistance and Home Program of the Ministry of Labor and Social Assistance. The social worker also contacted several of Margarita's family members who lived outside the community to determine if any of them could bring cooked food to Margarita on a daily basis.

The social worker and the family doctor obtained a reduction in the amount of money Margarita had to pay for medications at the polyclinic pharmacy and also arranged for Margarita to eat at a nearby cafeteria set up by the government to provide inexpensive meals for older persons with limited economic resources (Veitía Camejo & González Jubán, 2003). The social worker also contacted the Ministry of Labor and Social Assistance to request an increase in her deceased husband's social security pension to help pay for household expenses. The social worker, working with the family doctor, helped Margarita to obtain synthetic undergarments that Margarita had to wear because of her urinary incontinence, and to obtain other items that Margarita needed because of health problems.

Discussion and Conclusions

Barbara and Margarita's cases support our belief stated at the outset that the integration of social work into the health system of the community facilitates the social worker's access to a network of relationships among neighbors, health-care workers, and mass organizations capable of collective action to address the health and social problems of fragile older adults. Barbara and Margarita's examples illustrated how social workers' enhancement of social capital, including accessing the people's council and the Commission for the Prevention of Social Problems, helped two frail older adults continue to live in the community, despite their physical limitations. A communal ethos, defined earlier as popular participation of community residents and elected representatives in neighborhood social-action programs, also helped these two women. This communal ethos was evident in Margarita's doctor having shared his food with his patient, who was also his neighbor, and in the concern Barbara's neighbors expressed in Barbara's well-being.

The help that Barbara and Margarita received from their social workers resulted from an important link between the polyclinic and the community in Cuba. Barbara and Margarita's social workers functioned simultaneously as key EMAG team members at the municipal polyclinic and as community social workers with detailed knowledge about the neighborhood where their clients lived, because they spent afternoons working in the clinic. Barbara's social worker was able to find a substitute family for Barbara because of the worker's familiarity with Barbara's community and through the assistance of the empirical social worker. This example suggests the importance of close linkages between the polyclinic and the community in social work with the elderly.

Barbara's case also showed how the social worker was able to mobilize connections between institutions at the municipal, regional, and local levels, including the Municipal Office of the Ministry of Labor and Social Assistance (municipal level), the people's council (regional level), and the Commission for the Prevention of Social Problems (neighborhood level). The social worker was able to do this because of the close connection between polyclinics and municipal, regional, and local government offices and mass organizations. It is important to note the role of the state in the creation of these municipal, regional, and community institutions and the government's fostering of linkages among these entities to address the health and social needs of community members. Barbara's case illustrated how social capital in Cuba is embedded in relationships between institutions and community members that can benefit all those involved, making their work as a group more productive.

The case of Margarita showed that the social worker, interacting closely with the community doctor, helped Margarita obtain domestic

assistance, pay less for her medications, and eat for free at a local cafeteria established especially by the state for community members who
are poor. This working relationship between doctor and social worker
was facilitated by the contact that family doctors in Cuba have with
social workers on an ongoing basis in the polyclinic, as well as in the
community.

The examples illustrated in this chapter are also representative of
how social workers access social capital in work with the frail elderly
elsewhere in Cuba. Views about social workers' access of social capital
to aid the elderly must, however, remain tentative until further research
with a larger sample has been conducted. Nevertheless, others have
commented on the significance of social capital in promoting the well-
being of community members in various sectors of community life in
Cuba, including education (Carnoy, 2007), health care (Spiegel et al.,
2001), and community development (Uriarte, 2002).

What Can U.S. Social Workers Learn from
Their Cuban Counterparts?

The differences between Cuba and the United States may limit the
applicability of Cuba's community-oriented social work approach with
the frail elderly to gerontological social work in the United States. State-
generated social capital is usually the result of historical forces that are
country specific, such as the Cuban Revolution (Carnoy, 2007). Cuba's
"medicine in the community model" reflects a postrevolutionary socialist ideology and value system (Waitzkin, Iriat, Estrada, & Lamadrid,
2001), in a country where health care is free and universal. In Cuba, a
public-health approach is central to the delivery of health care, and
social work is embedded in the public-health system.

By contrast, the more individually oriented social work approach of
the United States may reflect the ideology and value system associated
with a capitalist economic system, in which the health-care system is
composed of a fragmented array of insurers and providers. U.S. health
care is characterized by costly medical services paid to a practitioner
who typically has little or no connection to the community ("A Health
System's 'Miracles,' " 2007). Individual consumers of health-care services
are encouraged to be independent of government support, which is why
public health plays a secondary role in U.S. health care.

Despite the differences between Cuba and the United States, Cuba's
social work approach can provide important insights for U.S. social
work educators, policy makers, and practitioners concerned with providing fragile, older community members with health and social services. It is important for gerontological social workers in the United

States to understand and know how to apply the concept of social capital when working with frail, elderly community members. Therefore, it may be useful for gerontological social workers in the United States to examine how Cuban social workers enhance social capital at the community level to provide services for the fragile elderly. U.S. social work practice with the elderly is increasingly carried out at the community level (Berkman, Silverstone, Simmons, Volland, & Howe, 2000), and U.S. social workers will continue to work in different types of community-based practice settings in the future (Crose & Minear, 1998). It is important for social workers in the United States to know how to access social relationships, ties, and networks among neighbors, community organizations, and health professionals in these different types of community settings.

The shift in gerontological social work in the United States from inpatient to outpatient and community-care settings is due, in part, to the growing influence of managed care and to the increased costs of institutional living (Berkman et al., 2000). It also reflects the federal government's preference for community-based care over institutional care, as stated in the 2001 Olmstead Act, Title III of Americans with Disabilities Act (National Institute on Disability and Rehabilitation Research, 2003). U.S. social workers are already involved in programs such as Project C.A.R.E., of the Administration on Aging, to help older persons to remain in their own homes for as long as possible and to avoid nursing home placement (Crose & Minear, 1998). Enhancing social capital, as Cuban social workers do, may be a cost-effective social work approach to helping the frail elderly in the community avoid institutionalization. Social work may be ideally suited to enhance social capital in this way (Kwok, 2003).

Growing numbers of persons in the United States will become old lacking caregiving family members (Conner, 2000). It is necessary to consider community-oriented models of care that can assist or even substitute for the family, as Cuba has done with its Substitute Family Program. The idea of finding "a substitute family" for the isolated older person may seem culturally alien and less than ideal to U.S. social workers who live in a society that is less community and family oriented than Cuba's. Nevertheless, it is important for U.S. social workers to find ways to help the elderly to remain in the community with their actual or fictive families, whenever possible. The promotion of foster home care for the frail elderly may be one way of doing so, although foster home care is not as yet widely accepted in the United States, nor is it currently a federally funded program (Oktay & Volland, 1987).

In Cuba, social work is integrated into the public-health system of the community, which facilitates social workers' access to sources of social capital. It may be useful for gerontological social work policy makers in the United States to consider ways that social workers at community clinics and hospitals can strengthen their ties with the communities in which their clients live, so as to enable them to access social capital to help their clients receive necessary health and social services.

The social work community in the United States faces tremendous challenges in preparing large numbers of social workers with the knowledge and the skills necessary to meet the needs of older Americans (Takamura, 2000). It is important that U.S. social work students who are interested in careers in gerontology learn community organizational and interdisciplinary team practice skills to help prepare them for service within communities and within interdisciplinary team settings, including health settings. The National Center of Geriatric Education Centers' curriculum on geriatrics now includes course material on these topics (U.S. Department of Health and Human Services, 2007). It is important to include modules in such a curriculum on how to access and work social capital in the community.

References

Águila, M. R., & Jubán, O. G. (2002). Familia sustituta e intervención social: Presentación de un caso. Paper presented at the Jornada Científica Anual de la Sociedad Cubana de Trabajadores Sociales de la Salud de la Provincia de la Ciudad de La Habana, Habana, Cuba, May 23, 2003.

A health system's "miracles" come with hidden costs. (2007, November 25). *The New York Times*, A4.

Alonso Galbán, P., Sansó Soberats, F. J., Díaz-Canel Navarro, A., Carrasco García, M., & Oliva, T. (2007, January). *Revista Cubana de Salud Pública*. Retrieved January 22, 2008, from http://www.scielosp.org

Arreola, G. (2008, January 12). Baja índice poblacional cubano en 2007 por segundo año consecutivo. *La Jornada*. Retrieved January 21, 2008, from http://www.jornada.unam.mx/2008/01/12

Berkman, B., Silverstone, B., Simmons, W. J., Volland, P. J., & Howe, J. L. (2000). Social work gerontological practice: The need for faculty development in the new millennium. *Journal of Gerontological Social Work, 34*(1), 5–23.

Bertera, E. M. (2003). Social services for the aged in Cuba. *International Social Work, 46*(3), 313–322.

Carnoy, M. (2007). *Cuba's academic advantage*. Stanford, CA: Stanford University Press.

Centro Iberoamericano de la Tercera Edad. (2005). SABE, proyecto salud, bienestar, y envejecimiento de los adultos mayores en América Latina y el Caribe (2000). Ciudad de La Habana, Cuba.

CEPAL. (2004). Política social y reformas estructurales: Cuba a principios del siglo XXI. Naciones Unidas. Retrieved January 25, 2007, from http://www.eclac.org

Conner, K. A. (2000). *Continuing to care: Older Americans and their families*. New York: Falmer Press.

Coyula, M., & Hamburg, J. (2004). Understanding slums: The case of Havana. Retrieved October 6, 2007, from the David Rockefeller Center for Latin American Studies Web site: http://www.drclas.harvard.edu

Creswell, J. W. (1994). *Qualitative and quantitative approaches.* Beverly Hills, CA: Sage Publications.

Crose, R., & Minear, M. (1998). Project CARE: A model for establishing neighborhood centers to increase access to services by low-income, minority elders. *Journal of Gerontological Social Work, 30*(3/4), 73–82.

Díaz-Briquets, S. (2002), The society and its environment. In R. A. Hudson (Ed.), *Cuba: A country study* (pp. 89–156). Washington, DC: Library of Congress.

Dilla, A. H. (1999). Cuba: virtudes e infortunios de la sociedad civil. *Revista Mexicana de Sociología, 61*(4), 129–148.

Dresang, L. T., Brebrick, L., Murray, D., Shallue, A., Sullivan-Vedder, L. (2005). Family medicine in Cuba: Community-oriented primary care and complementary and alternative medicine. *Journal of the American Board of Family Practice, 18*, 297–303.

Feinsilver, J. (1993). *Healing the masses: Cuban health politics at home and abroad.* Berkeley, CA: University of California Press.

Folland, S. (2007). Does "community social capital" contribute to population health? *Social Science and Medicine, 64*(11), 2342–2354.

Giraldo, G. (2007, June 10). Cuba's aging pains (and gains). *MEDICC* Review Cuba health reports. Retrieved January 21, 2007, from http://www.medicc.org/cubahealthreports/chr-article.php?&a=1031

Goicoechea-Balbona, A. M., & Conill-Mendoza, E. (2000). International inclusiveness: Publicizing Cuba's development of the "good life." *International Social Work, 43*(4), 435–451.

Kwok, J. (2003). Social welfare, social capital, and social work: Reflections of a Hong Kong social worker. Retrieved October 6, 2007, from http://www.lwb.gov.hk/download/services/events/040411_wel_forum/16_joseph_kwok_paper.pdf

Lochner, K., Kawachi, I., & Kennedy, B. P. (1999). Social capital: A guide to its measurement. *Health Place, 5*(4), 259–270.

Martínez Canals, E., & García Brigos, J. P. (2001). Comunidad y desarrollo: Una experiencia cubana en al área urbana. Cuba Siglo XX. Retrieved January 28, 2008, from http://www.nodo50.org/cubasigloXXI/politica/martinez1_310801.htm

MEDICC. (2007). Cuba health data. MEDICC Cuba health reports. Retrieved January 21, 2007, from http://www.medicc.org/cubahealthreports/

MEDICC. (2009). Cuba and the global health workforce: Health professionals abroad. Retrieved March 3, 2009, from http://medicc.org/ms/index.php.s=12&p=0

Midgeley, J., & Livermore, M. (1998). Social capital and local economic development: Implications for community social work practice. *Journal of Community Practice, 5*(1/2), 29–40.

National Institute on Disability and Rehabilitation Research. (2003). The Olmstead Act? What is it? Retrieved December 9, 2003, from http://www.worksupport.com/Archives/Olmstead.asp

Oficina Nacional de Estadísticas. (1998–1999). Anuario estadística de Cuba, 1996, 1997, 1999. Ciudad de La Habana, Cuba: ONE.

Oktay, J. S., & Volland, P. J. (1987). Foster home care for the frail elderly as an alternative to nursing home care: An experimental evaluation. *American Journal of Public Health, 77*(12), 1505–1510.

Pérez-Ávila, J. (2001). An overview of the Cuban health system with an emphasis on the role of primary health care and immunization. In L. Barberia & A. Castro (Eds.), (2002), *Seminar on the Cuban healthcare system: Its evolution, accomplishments and challenges* (pp. A9–12). David Rockefeller Center for Latin American Studies, Harvard University. Retrieved January 28, 2008, from http://www.medanthro.net/docs/castro_cuba.pdf

Poortinga, W. (2006). Social relations or social capital? Individual and community health effects of bonding social capital. *Social Science and Medicine, 63*(1), 255–270.

Program of Attention to Older Persons: An Interview (2000). *MEDICC Review.* Retrieved October 4, 2003, from http://www.medic.org/Medicc%20Review/I/aging/html/interview.html/

Rodríguez, V., Castellón, H., & Puga Gonzalez, D. (2004). *Características demográficas y socioeconómicas del envejecimiento de la población en España y Cuba.* Madrid, Spain: Consejo Superior de Investigaciones Científicas.

Roman, P. (2003). *People's power: Cuba's experience with representative government.* Lanham, MD: Rowman and Littlefield.

Spiegel, J., Bonet, M., Yassi, A., Mas, P., Tate, R., & Ibarra, A. (2001, October). *Social capital and health in Cuba: Case study of a community-based intervention program.* Paper presented at the 129th American Public Health Association Annual Meeting, Atlanta, Georgia.

Strug, D. (2004). An exploratory study in social work with older persons in Cuba. *Journal of Gerontological Social Work, 43*(2/3), 25–40.

Takamura, J. C. (2000). The aging of America and the older Americans act. In S. M. Kreiger, A. E. Fortune, & S. L. Witkin (Eds.), *Aging and social work: The changing landscapes* (pp. 127–136). Washington, DC: NASW Press.

Uriarte, M. (2002). *Cuba: Social policy at the crossroads: Maintaining priorities, transforming practice.* Boston, MA: Oxfam America.

U.S. Department of Health and Human Services (2007). Geriatric education centers. Retrieved January 19, 2008, from http://bhpr.hrsa.gov

Veitía Camejo, I., & González Jubán, O. (2003, September). *Análisis de los pacientes necesitados de servicio de alimentación identificados por el Departamento de Trabajo Social del Policlínico Ana Betancourt.* Paper presented at the III Encuentro Internacional de Trabajo Social Internacional, Habana, Cuba.

Waitzkin, H., Iriart, C., Estrada, A., & Lamadrid, S. (2001). Social medicine then and now: Lessons from Latin America. *American Journal of Public Health, 91*(10), 1592–1601.

Waller, J. (2002, Spring). Healing by primary intention. *Health Matters, 47*(2), 17. Retrieved January 1, 2007, from http://www.healthmatters.org.uk/issue47/primaryintention

PART IV

Mental Health

CHAPTER FOURTEEN

Mental-Health Care for Adolescents in Cuba

Susan E. Mason

"Love is such a profound human need that it is inconceivable that we should not construct our practice around encouraging its development."
—Dr. Elsa Gutierrez, child psychiatrist, Havana, Cuba

It is impossible to describe mental health treatment for adolescents in Cuba apart from the societal and ideological forces that permeate the country and bring about basic conflicts. The ideology of the 1959 Cuban Revolution focuses on freedom from oppression, the civic duty to help others, the prominence of the family unit, and the value of each citizen in the revolutionary process. It also supports the idea that there is wisdom in the country's revolutionary leaders; the ideas of Fidel Castro, Che Guevara, and José Martí are revered. For most Cubans, national identity includes the belief in the values of socialism and especially in the importance of sharing resources with all Cubans, regardless of background or education. The social system supports and reinforces what it calls "the ideas of the revolution" through centralization of most health services through the Ministry of Public Health (MINSAP), and education through the Ministry of Education (MINED).

Superimposed on these basic socialist beliefs are those of a growing number of adolescents and young adults who are calling for change.

These changes include but are not limited to accessibility to the Internet, lifting of travel restrictions, and the availability of more material goods. Only in the past year have cell phones and other electronics become available to those few Cubans who can pay for them; the younger generation wants increased access and more ways to raise their economic positions relative to the rest of the world.

Although most young Cubans agree that the values of the revolution are the foundation of modern Cuba, they are asking for less insulation. For young people and the mental-health providers who treat them for problems stemming from these conflicting values, the ideals of the revolution versus the wish for a more open and individualized society create conflict and confusion. While it is true that young people in most countries are vulnerable to rebellious and "acting out" behavior, the unique set of circumstances in Cuba makes these conflicts an important aspect of mental-health treatment.

It is important to understand the context in which young Cubans live, because it affects their mental health and treatment. A very large part of all mental-health care in Cuba is community based, owing to its theoretical grounding to sociology in addition to psychology and psychiatry. Mental-health care is free and mostly accessible to all Cuban adolescents. The extent to which these services are utilized by adolescents is, as in all countries, dependent on the perceived needs of young people and their families. The conflicts that Cuban adolescents experience that require mental-health interventions are often connected to their social environment and limitations imposed by the revolution.

The material in this chapter was taken from interviews with Cubans during several recent visits, and the limited number of published articles on mental health and young people in Cuba.

The Problem of "Double Morality"

"Double morality" in Cuba is defined as beliefs and behavior that both conform to the principles of the Cuban revolution and to the need for everyday survival (Prilleltensky, Sanchez Valdes, Rossiter, & Walsh-Bowers, 2002). Survival sometimes means that for economic reasons, people are forced to barter whatever goods they can acquire, legally or not, to obtain the necessities of life. For children and adolescents who are taught the strict values of the revolution in schools, this promotes a double message, or double morality. They see the neighborhood rituals of "taking home goods" and bartering them for needed groceries or extra food. Young people are then left to integrate these norms with what they learn in school. The effects of being exposed to two opposing sets of values have been identified by Cuban mental-health providers as potentially harmful for good adjustment to the Cuban way of life (Prilleltensky et al., 2002).

Double morality can also be seen in travel restrictions, access to computers, and access to transportation. Most Cubans cannot leave the country, and young people often want to understand why this is so. One young person interviewed said that the Cuban Constitution does not forbid him to travel, but visas must be applied for, and invariably they are denied to all but an elite few. He went on to say that he wanted to see what was beyond Cuba and that even though he loved his country, he felt constrained. Another young man said he wanted a computer or at least to use one to access the Internet. When asked why, he said, "Because everyone else in the world is doing it, so why can't we?" The growing tourist industry has brought more exposure to material goods, including clothing, cars, and a variety of electronic products. Increasingly, young people are participating in petty crimes targeted at tourists, and this too has fallen into the purview of clinicians taking care of young Cubans.

Setting the Stage: The Cuban Adolescent's Environment

There are many economically challenged countries in Latin America and in the world, but Cuba is unique in that it has a high literacy rate. The Cuban Ministry of Education claims the literacy rate to be 100 percent (United Nations Statistics Division, 2007). Most Cubans have graduated high school and large numbers have university degrees. All Cubans, regardless of their educational level, have difficulty finding housing in the cities, and food other than the sparse Cuban rations is difficult to obtain, as is clothing that most adolescents find acceptable. The adolescent boy or girl is likely to live in a small apartment or house with an extended family, which often includes a divorced couple who cannot split up because they have nowhere else to live. Parents may work full time but earn very little. Children are a cherished resource in Cuba, but adolescents see few options for economic success and creative expression.

University education is excellent for those who can pass the exams, and there are professional opportunities, especially in health care. Cuba's training of health-care providers is internationally recognized, but not every adolescent is so inclined or is able to be admitted to a medical school. Health-care providers are not economically better off than other professional workers, and in many cases they earn less. There is almost no access to recreational drugs, although alcohol can be obtained through illegal bartering, and religion is not part of most adolescents' lives. Most adolescents experiment with sex early on, but that can lead to consequences that many are not ready to face. This is the context in which to view adolescents in Cuba. It is also the environment that Cuban psychiatrists, psychologists, social workers, nurses, and other mental-health providers have themselves experienced.

The Development of Adolescent Psychiatry in Cuba

It is not surprising that in a country with scarce resources and a centralized health system, the development of a new field in mental-health treatment would initially be resisted. Traditionally in Cuba, as in many other countries, the pediatrician treated the child up until age eighteen, at which time the adult medical doctor or psychiatrist took over. Primary-care physicians and mental-health clinicians worked together as part of the Cuban Doctor and Nurse for the Family Program begun in 1984, to help coordinate services. Although many people saw a need for differentiating adolescents and older children from young children and from adults, leadership was needed to get the Ministry of Health to move in that direction. The person who stepped forward into the role of advocate for adolescent psychiatry was Dr. Elsa Gutierrez, a professor at the ELAM medical school in Havana and a practicing psychiatrist. Largely through her influence and her work with her students, the concept of a separate specialty took hold. The Adolescent Clinic in Havana was started and directed by Dr. Gutierrez until 2006, when she retired. At the clinic, special attention was paid to training that included psychiatrists, social workers, nurses, psychologists, and community workers. Many of these professionals went on to establish and work in similar clinics in other parts of the country.

Dr. Gutierrez promoted the overriding principle for the clinic: to intervene as early as possible and to include the family in treatment. Families were viewed as crucial because of housing shortages that almost guaranteed that adolescents would remain with their families for many years. The interactions between the adolescent and the rest of the family had to be considered in treatment and made positive. The Adolescent Clinic and similar clinics across the country offered day programs along with overnight facilities for young people in need of a respite. However, even when adolescents stayed overnight, select family members were encouraged to stay with them. The priority was, and still is, to keep families together as functioning units despite adolescents' behavior and/or symptoms.

Today, as dictated by Cuban law, if older children or adolescents need home care, parents can stay home and receive their full (or nearly full) salary from their jobs. This reduces the need for specialized residences and for most hospitalizations. The parent stays with the child, gets paid, and the family functions as the center of care. Social workers may look into the family home to ensure that the young patient is getting proper care, that medications are taken, and that appointments are kept. If there is a reason that families cannot assume this role, a caretaker is assigned to the home and paid for the work. At no time is the young patient without care. It is only in rare cases that the adolescent may be sent to one of the country's large psychiatric hospitals, and usually this is the case when there is severe noncompliance to care by the patients, when criminal activity takes place, or when there is repeated substance abuse.

The Concept of Love as an Intervention

In an interview with Dr. Gutierrez, she explained the concept of love as an intervention to promote healing. In this model, developed by Dr. Gutierrez, family members and especially the mother of a child with mental illness would be asked to attend separate sessions with the mental-health clinician. The focus of the family sessions would be to discuss the healing quality of love, and direct parents as to how to use it successfully. The principle behind this idea is that a child cannot develop normally without being given love, and that the clinician is no substitute for the parents. The family's ability to provide love for a child with a mental illness is enhanced by the availability of counseling and financial support.

In this model, the therapist's relationship with the adolescent and his or her family continues without time limitations and is not constrained by the family's ability to pay. In Cuba, all mental-health services are provided without charge. Clinicians are paid by the government, and the course of treatment depends on the judgment of the professionals. According to Dr. Guiterrez, most patients continue to see the same mental-health professionals throughout their treatment, and sometimes this may even extend to adulthood.

Love of children is an idea that is reinforced by Cuban culture. "Children are adored," explained a second prominent neuropsychiatrist trained in adolescent psychiatry interviewed at another time. "They are adored by the parents, the local community, and by the nation." Cuban culture focuses on solidarity that extends to neighbors taking responsibility for community children. It is not unusual, for example, for meetings with high-level government officials to have breaks where children are brought in to sing songs, dance, and so on. At such a meeting, where this author was present, government officials gave up their dour expressions, broke into smiles, and began to dance and sing along with the children. In this culture, it is understandable that the concept of love as a healing agent for all types of emotional and psychological problems has taken hold. Normative culture and the scarcity of many of the medications that are so commonly used in the United States have elevated love to the high status it enjoys as a healing intervention, especially with children and adolescents.

Identifying and Diagnosing Adolescent Psychological Problems

Identification of psychological problems for adolescents and older children comes about in Cuba in a number of ways. Parents may be distressed about a young person's behavior and speak with their family doctor, teachers may assess a student to be in need of help and refer him or her to a school social worker who in turn brings the student to the family doctor or polyclinic, the neighborhood clinic. There are Diagnostic and Assessment Centers in many parts of the country to supplement the work of the family doctors. Services are obtained at the polyclinic or at central clinics that specialize in adolescent service. When there are multiple problems such as substance abuse, sex and sexuality issues, and teenage pregnancy, young people are referred to specialized services. The specialized day clinics are mostly in the large cities. In the rural areas, teens may have to live in residences for part of the week because of the difficulty of obtaining transportation. Even so, the philosophy is the same, and efforts are made to keep young people and their families fully engaged.

Mental-health care for adolescents in Cuba, as with all health care in this country, is coordinated from a central office in the Ministry of Health (MINSAP) that maintains local offices throughout the country. Centralization has led Cuba to have a uniform and consistent protocol for care that extends from Havana into the outer districts.

For all diagnoses, the *Third Cuban Glossary of Psychiatry (GC-3)* is used (Otero-Ojeda, 2002). This adaptation of the *International Classification of Diseases (ICD)* was originally designed in 1975 to better reflect the realities of Cuban life. Key features include a strong emphasis on functioning, both personal and in school, and in occupations and with families. Also included are "normal" personality characteristics, such as the ability to make logical decisions, to be practical, and to conduct oneself "normally" in the area of romantic behavior. There is a section on managing needs, such as controlling hostility and indecisiveness. Finally, there is a miscellaneous section, where clinicians can add significant information that is not usually included in diagnostic protocols. Examples would be responses to therapeutic treatments, results of psychological reports, and social worker reports. Similar to the *Diagnostic and*

Statistical Manual of Mental Disorders (*DSM-IV*, American Psychiatric Association, 2000), there is room for medical conditions and environmental stressors, but clearly in the *GC-3* there is a stronger emphasis placed on the social aspect of patients than is typical in the United States.

As is true of the *DSM-IV*, Cubans used the advice and knowledge of prominent mental-health-care professionals in designing the *GC-3*. Because Cuba is a smaller country, with fewer mental-health professionals, a larger proportion of this group of professionals has had some say in the creation of the *GC-3*. Of course as with all health care in Cuba, mental health treatments driven by *GC-3* assessments need to conform to the policies of the centrally controlled health agencies.

There are several important aspects of the *GC-3* that specifically apply to young people and adolescents. They are childhood schizophrenia, generalized anxiety disorder of childhood, and neurotic mismanagement. There is also the category of risky consumption, behavior that refers to substance abuse by all ages but that is often found among younger people.

The Importance of Clinical Judgment in Treatment

In all Cuban psychological treatment, the clinician has a great deal of say, not only in treatment options but in diagnosis as well. Strict adherence to the categories in the *GC-3* or *ICD* is not necessarily considered good mental-health assessment. There are times when environmental factors such as family-relationship problems can influence the formal diagnosis. Good clinical judgment is considered just as important as a good "fit" into clinical categories. This of course can have both positive and negative effects on care. A young person who is lucky enough to be assigned to a competent, empathetic clinician may benefit from not being labeled early on in treatment, but not every health professional is equally skilled. It also leaves room for what has been called political diagnoses, which have been given to young people who were politically active against the government. Cuban mental-health workers consistently deny diagnosis used for this purpose, although indications of past use have been documented (Brown & Lago, 1991). This writer and others (Collinson & Turner, 2002) could find no data in support of the current use of political diagnoses in Cuba.

Overview of Mental-Health Practice with Children and Adolescents

Problems faced by parents of children and adolescents in Cuba are much the same as those in North America. They include learning problems, conflicts and rebellious behavior, and psychotic experiences. In Cuba there is less substance abuse than in the United States because there are fewer sources for illegal drugs, although alcohol is available. There are also fewer diagnoses of Attention Deficit Disorder (ADD) probably based on the cultural bias against using this label for young people and less availability of methylphenidate (Ritalin). Through increases in importations and manufacture in Cuba, more psychotropic medications are becoming accessible, and this has resulted in increases in prescription drug abuse by children and adolescents, as a way to get "high."

One problem that is prevalent among adolescents in the United States and largely nonexistent in Cuba is eating disorders. Cuban psychiatrists believe that Cuban culture's emphasis on health coupled with lack of a wide variety of foods inhibits this disorder from being widespread. Cuban adolescents do experience obsessions, anxieties, phobias, and of course depression, similar to adolescents in other parts of the world.

Child Abuse and Mental Health

Cuban children and adolescents can be both the perpetrators and victims of domestic violence and sexual abuse. The Cuban culture that strongly supports the prominence of the family calls on practitioners to make every effort to keep children in the home. In rare cases, when children are removed from their homes, they are usually placed with close relatives. In-home counseling is commonplace when there are suspected cases of child abuse. Clinicians may be alerted to abuse problems by teachers, community physicians, or after-school activity counselors. Once this occurs, a community social worker may do a preliminary investigation followed by a referral to a clinical social worker, a psychologist, or a child psychiatrist. In-home evaluations allow clinicians to see the whole picture, and families are subjected to enormous community pressure to allow home interventions. In Cuba, children are viewed as members of a community, and neighbors take an interest in all the children in the surrounding area. This is true in the rural districts as well as the cities. It is also true that the government encourages neighborhood monitoring as a way to ensure that children get the most care with the smallest expenditure of resources. Juvenile correctional facilities, foster care homes, and orphanages are kept at an absolute minimum and in some areas are nonexistent.

Cuban mental-health professionals are concerned that in a culture that emphasizes the privacy of sexuality and where family shame is to be avoided at all costs, there are too many coverups of incidents that require intervention. A child psychiatrist in Havana stated: "We need to do more. We cannot be as silent as we have been about child abuse. If we knew more, we could do more in the way of prevention through community education and early interventions."

A study of child-abuse victims in Havana between 1990 and 1991 found that more females than males were abused (163 to 46) and that 156 were under age twelve and 53 were between twelve and fifteen years of age (Castro Espín, Córdova Llorca, & Bardisa Escurra, 2004). In this study, there were none of the usual physical marks of child abuse on the victims, indicating either a one-time event or a concerted effort toward keeping abuse a secret. Most of the victims came from families where physical punishment of children was common, but there were no reported cases of revictimization. Such data are difficult to interpret without further information, but it appears that once children and adolescents were abused, there was a family-based intervention that stopped the abuse. Since removing children from families is rare in Cuba, it may be that the abuser was removed or that the family received counseling, or both.

Prevention as a Way of Life

A psychosocial approach to child and adolescent mental-health care is taken at every stage of symptom and function disability. The idea behind the model is to identify the problem as early as possible. For example, if a child is beginning to express thoughts or behave in a way that is of concern to teachers or community workers, he or she may be directed to join a community program where behavior is monitored. Many community programs that involve music and art are encouraged by a Cuban culture that holds these endeavors in high esteem. It is likely that many children with the beginnings of what we would term Attention Deficit Disorder (ADD), burn off excess energy in artistic programs and sports that are carefully structured for such children. These programs are available in most neighborhoods in Havana and are overseen by the community liaison person connected to the government and the Communist Party. Although this might sound ominous to those in the United States, for most Cubans, party officials are viewed as resources for obtaining additional funded projects from the government. They are generally representatives from the Committees for the Defense of the Revolution (CDRs), government-supported organizations, and are popular in neighborhoods for promoting pro-active public-health policies acceptable to most Cubans. In one illustrative case, a fourteen-year-old was judged by the community physician to need psychological counseling based on her disruptive behavior and signs of depression. A referral was made to the local polyclinic, and the CDR representative was informed. The girl was helped to keep her counseling appointments through the CDR representative's efforts in obtaining transportation and reminding the family of the importance of treatment. In this case, as in most, the well-being of the child became a community concern; the family was expected to fully cooperate with the girl's treatment.

Sex and Sexuality

Like everything else in Cuba, the government has a central role in setting policies regarding sex education and resources devoted to the promotion of healthy sex and sexuality. The Ministry of Education (MINED) writes and monitors the sex education program presented in all Cuban schools. The program consists of in-class instruction and extracurricular activities that often involve parents. Classes and activities take place at the elementary-school level right through to the university classes. Television broadcasts targeted at adolescents include short films on responsible sexual behavior, sponsored by the Ministry of Public Health (MINSAP) and the National Center for Sex Education (CENESEX). Community-intervention programs and counseling centers that specialize in helping to promote responsible sexual behavior are set up throughout the country. One goal that has been successfully met is the reduction of drop-out rates due to pregnancy and marriage. Its effectiveness is demonstrated by a reduction from 1,038 to 240 dropouts between 1997 and 1998 and 2000 and 2001. Cubans also claim that early sexual relations in Cuba among adolescents have decreased from about 30 percent to about 10 percent (Torres Cuerto, 2004).

In Cuba, as in most countries today, young people often experiment with sex. Age of experimentation may depend on the home environment, with the earlier ages more often associated with family dysfunctions such as divorce, imprisonment, and use of drugs, according to Cuban writers. During later adolescence, sexual behavior becomes more common, and with few Cuban male adolescents using condoms, pregnancy and sexually transmitted diseases become a risk (Guerrero, 2004).

Having sexual relations is not necessarily a reason to need counseling, but it can lead to emotional states that require intervention, especially if the sex does not involve a lasting relationship. Homosexual and bisexual behaviors are legally tolerated in that there are no laws that prohibit homosexuality. On the other hand, there are no written legal protections, and undoubtedly there are numerous incidents of discrimination, especially in the provinces away from Havana. Cuban law specifically states that marriage is between a man and a woman, but in Havana, Santiago, and other large cities, many gay and lesbian couples live together and function as a family unit (Castro Espín & Abreu Guerra, 2004). Nevertheless, young people who are homosexual or who think they might be, can get supportive counseling. The same is true for adolescents who have gender diversity or transgender issues (Rodríguez Lauzerique & Bravo Fernández, 2004).

Medication

The availability of psychotropic medication has improved over the last decade, but it remains a problem. Cuba's pharmaceutical industry does produce psychotropic medications, but dose sizes are limited and many drugs that are used commonly in other parts of the world are not readily available. For example, the older medications for depression (the tricyclics) are used because they are available through less-expensive importation from countries other than the United States. Ritalin, or methylphenidate, is produced in Cuba but only in limited doses. Although Cuban psychiatrists have by world standards excellent medical training, they may not be experienced in using the newer medications because of the lack of availability.

Young people are less inclined to take medications with side effects that many of the older drugs are known to have, and that makes medication compliance a problem. Child psychiatrists know this and some use it as a rationale for avoiding prescribing medications when possible. Instead they rely on the resources of the watchful community, promote interventions that include families, and use the generous social services provided by the government.

Protecting Youth from Outside Influences: An Ethical Dilemma

A dilemma surrounding the psychological care of adolescents concerns the influence of the tourist industry that is supported by the government to bring in needed hard currencies. Mental-health workers find it difficult to counsel young people to reject the material goods tourists bring to Cuba, when most Cubans, including the clinicians, would like more of these government-prohibited items. The increase in the tourist industry has resulted in increased exposure to the outside way of life. A recent study conducted in resort areas outside of Havana reported that Cuban youth are now expressing interest in working in the tourist industry, as they get a glimpse of the outside world. At the same time, these young people risk exposure to the underside of tourism that includes petty crime, gambling, drugs, and prostitution (Spiegel et al., 2007). Local communities have responded by creating youth-centered programs supported and funded by the central government. Data on the effectiveness of these programs in keeping young people safe from the corruption of tourism are not available, and certainly this is not a new problem in the Caribbean countries. It is new, however, for Cuba in that tourism promotion has only been encouraged since the 1990s, when the economy severely declined because of the withdrawal of funding from and subsequent fall of the Soviet Union. Reforms instituted by Raúl Castro allow Cubans to stay in tourist hotels, and although this will not affect most young people, who have limited resources, it may enable young Cubans to more easily meet and talk with young people from other countries.

Conclusion

Recent reforms in Cuba indicate that the country may be approaching a transitional phase in which some of the aspects of the mental-health system are likely to change. Resources currently devoted to providing young people and families with unlimited, free care may be diverted, resulting in a system less dependent on human capital and more on technology. When Cuba obtains more psychotropic medications, the newly trained psychiatrists are likely to use them. Less emphasis may be placed on sociological methods of community interventions and psychological counseling for families. What is likely not to change is Cuba's love for its children and the cultural belief that all people are entitled to the dignity that comes from good, accessible health care, including mental-health care.

References

American Psychiatric Association. (2000). *Diagnostic and statistical manual of mental disorders* (4th ed., text rev.) Washington, DC: Author.

Brown, C. J., & Lago, A. M. (1991). *The politics of psychiatry in revolutionary Cuba.* New Brunswick, NJ: Transaction Publishers.

Castro Espín, M., & Abreu Guerra, E. (2004). Homoerotic, homosexual, and bisexual behaviors. In R. T. Francoeur & R. J. Noonan (Eds.), *The Continuum complete international encyclopedia of sexuality* (p. 270). New York: The Continuum Publishing Group.

Castro Espín, M., Córdova Llorca, M. D., & Bardisa Escurra, L. (2004). Child sexual abuse. In R. T. Francoeur & R. J. Noonan (Eds.), *The Continuum complete international encyclopedia of sexuality* (pp. 270–271). New York: The Continuum Publishing Group.

Collinson, S. R., & Turner, T. H. (2002). Not just salsa and cigars: Mental health care in Cuba. *Psychiatric Bulletin, 26,* 185–188.

Guerrero, N. (2004). Adolescents. In R. T. Francoeur & R. J. Noonan (Eds.), *The Continuum complete international encyclopedia of sexuality* (pp. 266–267). New York: The Continuum Publishing Group.

Otero-Ojeda, A. A. (2002). Third Cuban glossary of psychiatry (GC-3): Key features and contributions. *Psychopathology, 35,* 181–184.

Prilleltensky, I., Sanchez Valdes, L., Rossiter, A., & Walsh-Bowers, R. (2002). Applied ethics in mental health in Cuba: Part II—Power differentials, dilemmas, resources, and limitations. *Ethics & Behavior, 12*(3), 243–260.

Rodríguez Lauzerique, M., & Bravo Fernández, O. (2004). Gender diversity and transgender issues. In R. T. Francoeur & R. J. Noonan (Eds.), *The Continuum complete international encyclopedia of sexuality* (p. 270). New York: The Continuum Publishing Group.

Spiegel, J. M., González, M., Cabrera, G. J., Catasus, S., Vidal, C., & Yassí, A. (2007, December, 14). (E-publication ahead of print). Promoting health in response to global tourism expansion in Cuba. *Health Promotion International.* Retrieved January 13, 2008, from http://www.liu.xplorex.com/?p2=/modules/liu/publications/view.jsp&id=2074

Torres Cuerto, G.M.A. (2004). Government policies and programs. In R. T. Francoeur & R. J. Noonan (Eds.), *The Continuum complete international encyclopedia of sexuality* (pp. 264–265). New York: The Continuum Publishing Group.

United Nations Statistics Division. (2007). Millennium development goal indicators. Retrieved on April 21, 2008, from http://mdgs.un.org/unsd/mdg/Search.aspx?q=literacy%20Cuba

CHAPTER FIFTEEN

Mental-Health Care and Concerns in Cuba

Susan E. Mason

"People become crazy depending on how they have lived."
—Dr. Raúl Gil Sanchez, Psychiatrist, Regla, Cuba

Mental-health care in Cuba is based on a community model wherein the community participates in creating programs that support good mental health. Mental-health services are part of Cuba's national health system and are under the supervision of the Ministry of Public Health (MINSAP). Mental-health care in Cuba combines environmental interventions, psychological counseling, and medications. Environmental interventions, which can be thought of as sociological, take the form of symptom prevention and control through encouraging families to be supportive, community members to get involved, and offering programs with constructive activities. Psychological treatments take the form of cognitive and family therapy models. Clinicians are mainly psychologists, with additional work being performed by psychiatrists, social workers, and nurses. Mental-health clinicians receive both formal discipline-specific training at schools and universities and exposure to new psychotherapy techniques at national and international conferences held on the island. Psychiatrists prescribe medication and are assisted by psychiatric nurses. Cuban psychiatrists accomplish a great deal with the few medications that are available, such as the older generation of antidepressants and antipsychotic drugs. The United States embargo on Cuba prohibits many of the larger pharmaceutical companies from selling medications to Cuba.

This chapter presents a view of the mental-health system with a focus on unique Cuban strengths and continuing challenges. It addresses the structure of the system and the concerns that continue to confront Cubans today. It is based on both published sources and the author's experiences from multiple visits to Cuba. Data from observations and formal and informal meetings with Cubans about their mental-health system form the basis of the information presented.

Community Interventions as Treatment

Community interventions are structured to achieve two goals: prevention and containment. The Cuban mental-health system closely follows primary prevention strategies that aim to prevent an illness, and secondary prevention strategies that aim to keep the first signs of illness from becoming a full-blown syndrome as outlined by Caplan (1964). Cuban mental-health strategists accomplish primary and secondary prevention by carefully planning programs that are implemented by local community groups such as the Committee for the Defense of the Revolution (CDR) and the Federation of Cuban Women (FMC). These mental-health programs carried out by the CDR and FMC are approved and funded by the centralized agency responsible for public health and health care in Cuba, MINSAP.

Primary Prevention in the Community

Primary prevention programs in Cuban communities include good prenatal care that monitors mothers' health and habits such as nutrition and intake of alcohol, good obstetric care to prevent organic brain injuries, and well-baby programs that ensure adequate nutrition and treatment for infectious diseases. In Cuba, all pregnant women and mothers are encouraged to adhere to rules of good care; if they do not, they can be encouraged to live in group homes for pregnant mothers. The family doctor and the FMC cooperate in finding the best solution for noncompliant women. According to a high-placed public-health official (personal communication), most Cubans agree that the well-being of the baby is so important that the mother needs to comply with good care. Taking good care of children before and immediately after birth is one assertive way that the Cuban health system tries to prevent a long list of illnesses including those that affect the brain. Another is to discourage people who are diagnosed with a severe mental illness from having children. Although there are no laws that demand sterilization or abortions for this group, families are often convinced that this is the correct option for family members with schizophrenia or another severe and persistent mental illness.

For older children and adolescents, primary prevention programs consist of after-school talk groups, sports activities, and music and art programs that children are strongly encouraged to join. The rationale for these programs is to keep young people busy so that depression, anxiety, and behavior problems do not develop. Young people are encouraged to participate in school and community groups that discuss and address conflicts within their families. These groups are not just for children that display problematic behavior; they are for large numbers of children (if not all in each primary and secondary school) and are meant to prevent future problems. Some communities have started antidrug groups for young people in anticipation of the negative effects of tourism that brings exposure to people from outside of Cuba (Spiegel et al., 2007).

Health promotion, a concept that originated in the 1970s in Canada and was adopted by the World Health Organization, views health as a resource that requires careful development. Conceptually, health promotion focuses on the environment, biology, and available health care (Donaldson & Donaldson, 1994; Greene, 2003). Cuba was quick to utilize this concept, first in its movement toward universal health care that began to demonstrate success in the 1970s, and later in the inclusion of psychological well-being in the health-promotion philosophy. The concept of environment as a health resource worked well in the Cuban social and political system; it mobilized neighborhoods to take care of its people, and it promoted the perception of a caring government. People were asked to sacrifice privacy and accept the political responsibility of health promotion, which included mental health. The payoff was to be an inclusive health/mental-health system that was both free and effective.

Secondary Prevention

Secondary prevention strategies are in place for people who are diagnosed with a mental illness or who are exhibiting behavior that may be a precursor to a diagnosis. For serious mental illnesses, examples of secondary prevention would be to identify and contain the early premorbid symptoms before they develop into a full-blown syndrome (McGorry & Jackson, 1999; Warner, 2001).

The Community Mental-Health Center

Community Mental-Health Centers (CMHCs) are located throughout the country and serve both patients and their families. Patients typically live at home and come to the center on a daily basis. In most cases, the patient is free to come as often or as infrequently as he or she likes. Occasionally, the center staff recommends that a patient come on a regular basis, and staff members go to a patient's home to encourage attendance. The family doctor or a member of the CDR or the FMC can place pressure on families to ensure center attendance for someone judged in need. This is how the Cuban revolutionary ideology, that each citizen is obligated to make his or her best effort to remain healthy, works to involves communities to care for each member. Today, it appears that most Cubans agree that community intervention in matters pertaining to mental health is necessary and helpful to identified patients and their families.

Activities for patients at the CMHC include participation in talk-therapy groups that are largely based on a cognitive model; art and music therapy groups; scheduled visits with doctors and nurses as needed; and activities that are geared to individuals' abilities and preferences, such as horticulture, basketweaving, poetry writing, and active sports. Patient groups often take walks in the community and go on field trips.

In most Community Mental Health Centers there are efforts to reach out to the communities, especially to the caregivers of patients. In Guanabacoa, a western suburb of Havana, the CMHC staff invite caregivers to regular meetings to discuss feelings of stress or depression related to their caregiver role. In many cases, the caregiver becomes an occasional CMHC patient to help the caregiver cope with the difficulties of the caregiver role. Caregivers sometimes phone CMHC staff at their homes or even knock on their doors in the evenings and on holidays when they may be feeling overwhelmed or experiencing a patient-initiated crisis. Family members caring for people with mental illness know they will get help even in the after hours. CMHC staff are dedicated to their work, but they report sometimes feeling stressed by being on call twenty-four hours a day. In the words of one staff member who lives in the community: "This is what we do, but of course it is stressful for us too. I could be having dinner with my family and I get a call. Then I go. I have even had people knock on my door and I have to stop everything I am doing."

The importance of family values, coupled with the housing shortage in Cuban cities, means that most patients with severe mental illnesses live with their families, often in crowded apartments. Patients with ongoing psychoses or unresponding depressions are understandably difficult for many families to manage. Family members may apply to the Rehabilitation Office of the Ministry of Public Health for full-time salaries to stay home and care for their ill family member. Part-time income may be granted to families when the patients attend the CMHC. These compensatory programs alleviate financial stresses in many families. The outreach services of the CMHCs provide both primary and secondary prevention services in that they address the needs of the whole family, the well members and the identified patients.

The Role of the Family Doctor in Mental-Illness Prevention

Family doctors are currently responsible for about two hundred families in a neighborhood. During the past several years, there have been doctor shortages due to the government policy of encouraging young doctors to spend several years abroad working in poor areas, mostly in Latin America. The "doctors for oil" program, sending doctors to Venezuela in exchange for oil, is an example of such a program, but Cuban doctors also serve where there are no immediate tangible benefits except for goodwill for Cuba.

A question that many family doctors face is the extent to which they are expected to serve as community monitors as part of their medical responsibilities. Ideologically, mental illness falls within the principle that it is the duty of each citizen to be as healthy as possible. This means that aberrant behavior becomes a reportable problem that warrants intervention. The problem that family doctors often contend with is that apparent symptoms and functioning behaviors can be interpreted in many ways and are not easily assessed as pathology. In Cuba, the assessment tool used to diagnose mental illnesses is the *Third Cuban Glossary of Psychiatry* (*GC-3*), an adaptation of the *International Classification of Diseases* (*ICD*) (Otero-Ojeda, 2002). In this diagnostic tool, there is a strong emphasis on everyday functioning, thinking logically, controlling anger, and normative behavior. Cuban medical doctors are expected to report unusual or disruptive behavior to a representative of the CDR, who in turn sends a community worker to the home to make a further assessment. If the person whose behavior is in question is thought to need treatment, he or she is referred for professional assessment by a mental-health clinician, usually a psychologist.

The presentation of clear-cut symptoms, as outlined in the *GC-3* and the *ICD*, bring about little conflict for community doctors; they are glad the patient will get appropriate treatment. Aberrant behavior, however, can be more problematic. Family doctors are challenged to consider the effects of diversity, culture, and religion as well as the preferences and resources of the family. The doctor is aware that mental-health referral may place the person's job in jeopardy or bring about stigma to family members. This again addresses the role of the family doctor and his or her place within the context of Cuban society. The position that "health is a social responsibility," expressed by a psychiatrist in Cuba, is modified by the family doctor's knowledge of the community and the possible outcomes of such referrals.

The Polyclinic

Polyclinics serve several neighborhoods in the cities and in rural areas. Many smaller towns and villages may share one clinic. Counseling and psychological care are included in the large array of medical, rehabilitation, and dental services available at the polyclinics. Mental-health patients are referred by family doctors, social workers, or psychologists working at schools or in community diagnostic centers, or they may simply walk in themselves and ask for an appointment. Since all medical and psychological services in Cuba are free and open to all people, there are no insurance or payment issues. Clinician availability and transportation to the polyclinic are the only obstacles that a "walk-in" patient must face. Polyclinic mental-health staff assess the patient and schedule appointments or make a referral to a CMHC, depending on the severity of the problem and the patient's ability to travel. There may be a referral to a Grandparent's Club, a day program for older persons, some of whom may be suffering from cognitive impairments.

Depending on where the polyclinic is located, the biggest problem affecting access today is transportation. Although there has been improvement in public transportation in the last several years, it remains inadequate and the average person does not have access to a car. For people with psychological problems, negotiating infrequent and crowded buses may be beyond their abilities. Soliciting rides from private cars, a common practice in Cuba, may be too frightening for people with a variety of mental illnesses. Missed appointments are frequent, and transportation issues are often the cause.

The Psychiatric Hospital

The psychiatric hospital is available for individuals who cannot be managed at home. Psychiatric units are attached to many medical hospitals, and most admissions are voluntary. The typical stay in these units is less than thirty days. There are seven specialized psychiatric hospitals that largely house long-term patients, although these also have outpatient and short-term facilities. Patients who have no homes or families willing to take them back can remain in the specialized hospitals. People with chronic and severe schizophrenia make up most of the residents, but there are also patients with various forms of dementia, nonresponsive depression, addictions, and forensic diagnoses. Treatments include cognitive therapy, medications, electroconvulsive therapy (ECT), and music and art classes. The seven psychiatric hospitals throughout Cuba vary in their physical facilities and treatment resources, but they are similar in philosophy; they exist for those who cannot function in the community (Kates, 1987; Skaine, 2003). Over the past decade, most psychiatric hospitals have made a concerted effort to reduce the number of patients.

Cuba's largest psychiatric hospital, Hospital Psiquiátrico de la Habana (informally known as Mazorra), is on the outskirts of Havana, and has between 3,000 and 3,500 patients. According to an administrator, the goal is to reduce the number of patients to a thousand, but this has not yet occurred. Patients come to the hospital on their own, through the outpatient facility, or from the polyclinics. Sometimes families bring in a relative who has a history of mental illness and is displaying behavior problems in the home. Police bring in forensic patients such as illegal drug users, people convicted of sex crimes, perpetrators of family violence, and those exhibiting other types of criminal behavior. Forensic patients live in locked units, wear pajamas, and participate in carefully watched, structured activities. The nonforensic patients wear street clothes and appear to have mobility within the facility. The nonmandated patients are free to leave. Leaving, however, is difficult if families are unwilling or pressured by their community CDR not to take them back. In Cuba, where the housing shortage is acute, if patients cannot return to their families, they have limited options. People need money, shelter, food ration books, and health care, and they cannot get them without local government approval, usually through the community CDR councils. Although there are a number of protected dormitories throughout the country for homeless people, and foster families care for patients who cannot return to their own homes, these resources are scarce and require approval by the hospitals and health bureaucracies. According to an administrator at the hospital, sometimes patients elope but they invariably return on their own or are brought back by family members. The average length of stay is twenty-eight to thirty days for acute cases and three to four months for chronic patients.

One function of the psychiatric hospitals is to rehabilitate people with addictions, and many of these patients are held involuntarily. In Cuba, illegal drug use and addictions are in conflict with the health-promotion ideology of the government. Cuba has a very strict antidrug policy and drug dealing by Cubans is punished with long prison terms and even death. The Cuban government's position is that people with illegal drug addictions are dangerous to the health of the country. There are no public-opinion surveys on this or any government policy, but from informal questioning by the author, it appears that most people agree. People sent to the psychiatric hospitals for drug-related behavior must demonstrate complete rehabilitation before they can leave.

Alcohol abuse is far more prominent than abuse of illegal drugs, and for most Cubans alcohol is by far easier to obtain. There is a saying in Cuba that people will drink until the last drop is gone. This may be true, in part, because alcohol must be purchased with hard currency, and the next drink may be difficult to obtain. Many Cubans do have hard currency from working in the tourist industry or from bartering gifts received from relatives in the United States and elsewhere. There is also an illegal alcohol trade in Cuba, which, combined with the availability of hard currency, gives most people some degree of access. In most cases, alcohol abuse is treated at the polyclinic level, but in certain cases, hardcore drinkers who cannot be managed by their families are brought to the psychiatric hospital to dry out.

There are indications that in the past, both pre- and post-1959, political prisoners and dissidents have been held against their will in Cuba's psychiatric hospitals, but it is not clear that this misuse of psychiatry continues (Collinson & Turner, 2002). Allegations of psychiatric abuse are difficult to verify because information is not available to visitors. *The Cuban Criminal Code* states that anyone who "breaks the rules of social co-existence or disturbs the order of the community, . . . is considered to be socially dangerous by virtue of such anti-social conduct." (Inter American Commission on Human Rights, 1997). The extent to which Cuban psychiatric hospitals are used as prisons or worse, as place for psychic torture, is not generally known, although such accusations can be found on the Internet (*Medicina Cubana*, 2006).

The Mental Health Professions

It is estimated that there are approximately 1,100 psychiatrists, 1,000 psychologists, 300 psychiatric nurses, and 1,400 psychiatric social workers in Cuba to serve a population of more than eleven million people (World Health Organization, 2005). Master's-level psychologists do the bulk of the mental-health counseling in the polyclinics. Psychiatrists prescribe medication and conduct neurological examinations. Nurses monitor the health of the psychiatric patients and help in distributing medications and other needed supplies. Social workers mostly perform case management for psychiatric patients. Social workers visit families, hold family meetings, and assess the patient's environment to ensure access to services and benefits. If a patient is disabled for psychological reasons, he or she is not expected to work and still receives food and clothing rations. Social workers set up these and other entitlements such as the right of a family caregiver to remain at home with a patient who is in need of home care. The family caregiver receives a full or half government salary, depending on how many hours they deliver care to the patient in the home. Social workers are less likely to conduct psychotherapy, leaving that task to the psychologists.

Psychiatrists work mostly in community mental-health centers, medical hospitals that have psychiatry units, specialized diagnostic and treatment centers such as the Adolescent Treatment Center in Havana, and in the psychiatric hospitals. They perform a variety of services that includes psychotherapy, medication management, diagnostic and assessment work, and supervision of psychologists. Additionally, they work in public-health programs designing and implementing primary and secondary preventive strategies. They may be clinic directors and often are involved, along with psychologists, in conducting outcome research. Social workers are typically not included in research activities, but this may change because of shortages of psychiatrists and psychologists.

The Mariel Boatlift

The Mariel boatlift is well known in Cuban-U.S. relations as a time when large numbers of Cubans, many of whom were released from psychiatric hospitals, were allowed to emigrate to the United States. The museum display at the Mazorra psychiatric hospital outside of Havana shows boats filled with ex-patients leaving for Florida. The exhibit description portrays this as a means of freeing up beds in that facility. The extent to which the psychiatric patients affected the social structure of Florida is not entirely clear, but there is evidence that there was only a minor impact on Florida's economy (Card, 1989).

In 1980, ten thousand Cubans stormed the Peruvian Embassy in Havana in an attempt to gain asylum. A series of events propelled mostly by difficult economic conditions led Fidel Castro and then U.S. President Jimmy Carter to allow about 125,000 Cubans to emigrate to the United States. Cuban-American exiles arranged for the boats that left from the Cuban port of Mariel between April and October of 1980. It soon became known that many of the émigrés had been prisoners and patients at psychiatric hospitals. The U.S. government stopped receiving the Cuban émigrés because of the large number of people, the negative publicity about the source of many of the émigrés, and the unwillingness to accept people from other countries such as Haiti. The decision to "empty" the psychiatric hospitals during the Mariel boatlift was said to be the Cuban government's way of saving the expense of caring for thousands of patients. Cuban mental-health professionals helped patients get ready for the journey, but the decision to encourage the exodus was made by the government, not the clinicians.

Suicide—A Prominent Problem in Cuba

Cuba has a high rate of suicide when compared to similar countries in the Caribbean. The suicide rate in 2004 was 13.5 per 100,000 (20.3 per 100,000 for males and 6.6 for females). The only Latin American country with a higher suicide rate was Uruguay with 15.1. The rate for the United States is listed as 11.1 per 100,000 people (World Health Organization, 2007). It is difficult to know why the suicide rate is so high, but Luis Perez Jr., who wrote the landmark book on the subject, *To Die in Cuba*, claims that the history of worker abuse and a culture that accepts suicide as a way out explains the phenomenon (Perez Jr., 2005). The depression that often precedes suicidal behavior can be treated at the polyclinics and the CMHCs, but as in many other countries, mental-health services are not always utilized. The fact that in Cuba there is no charge for services doesn't seem to matter. Other explanations for the high suicide rate may include the volatility of the economy, the growing tourist industry that contrasts the conditions that Cubans live under with that of other countries, and the disappointment of underemployment fueled by a high literacy rate.

In the past, young women were more likely to take their own lives than young men during times of severe economic stress, such as the 1990s, after the Soviet Union terminated its economic support. The World Health Organization data from 1996 showed that in the age range of fifteen to nineteen, young Cuban women committed suicide at a rate of more than twice that of men (12.5 to 6.1 per 100,000) (Wasserman, Cheng, & Jiang, 2005). These numbers have since reversed. In 2004, at every age, males were more likely to commit suicide, and between 1995 and 2004 the rate for women declined by 56 percent and for males by only 21 percent. (World Health Organization, 2007). During this time period, the Cuban economy markedly improved, but only further research can supply an explanation for this change. It is interesting, however, that one study reported that Cuban women with the diagnosis of schizophrenia expressed less satisfaction in their quality of life than men (Vandiver, 1998). Again, it is difficult to know how to interpret this, but it may be that depression is linked to the volatility of the economy, and women may suffer more when there are fewer resources. The response of the government is to continue the primary prevention programs that target vulnerable groups, especially in areas where high concentrations of tourist activities show Cubans to be economically disadvantaged (Spiegel et al., 2007).

Note: The problem of suicide was never mentioned to this author on four recent trips to the island.

Stigma and Mental Health

"Sure there is stigma. It may not be outright, but people are ashamed that a family member is not quite right in the head."
(a Cuban clinician)

The almost universal prejudice against people with mental illness is alive and well in Cuba. Families may try to mask the problem by declaring that the person in question drinks too much, an affliction that is more widely acceptable than if that person were depressed, manic, or delusional. Housing shortages result in most people with mental illness remaining with their families, according to interviews with Cuban social workers and psychologists. Vandiver (1998) reported that in her sample of twenty-seven Cubans with schizophrenia, five lived alone and twenty-two lived either with parents or spouses. She also found that most (fifteen) had never married; that was a slightly higher percentage than a comparison group in the United States. The sample in this study was small, and these statistics only show us an indirect picture of how people with schizophrenia live in Cuba. The extent to which families and people with the various mental illnesses are discriminated against is difficult for visitors to assess. Cuban law guarantees all people who are disabled full economic benefits, and their families get benefits as well.

Community Mental Health Centers sponsor outreach programs that focus on providing psychoeducation to community members, especially those who provide neighborhood services, such as barbers, bus drivers, and other people who may come into contact with people with mental illness. These programs aim to reduce prejudices and combat many people's irrational fears of those with psychiatric histories. They also encourage community tolerance and support for families having identified patients living at home. There are no available data on the effectiveness of these efforts, but according to one psychologist, much more needs to be done.

An ameliorating factor to the prevalence of stigma in Cuba is the widespread appreciation for art and music. If a person diagnosed with a mental illness is talented in these areas, he or she is less likely to experience discrimination. This is especially true when tourists appreciate the art or music of the person with a mental illness, as this may translate into additional family income. In Cuba, people sell art works and music CDs on the street and at art fairs. Additionally, today's Cuban economy has more workers than jobs, and because disabled patients and their families are often entitled to benefits, people who cannot work are not an economic burden. Nevertheless, Cuban clinicians affirm the stigma attached to having a mental illness that affects patient's social relations. Vandiver (1998) describes the difficulty that women with schizophrenia had in establishing social relationships, in her study at an outpatient clinic at the Mazorra hospital. Men reported friendships among the other patients, but neither gender mentioned community-based relationships.

Medications

"Please bring in [from the U.S.] as many psychotropic medications as you can. We collect from everyone and use them when they are needed for patients." (a Cuban psychiatrist)

"If I have to make a decision about purchasing life-saving antibiotics or psychotropic medications, the choice is clear." (official in Office of Public Health)

There are psychotropic medications in Cuba, but selections and doses are limited. Most of the medication for treating mental illnesses are first- and second-generation drugs and not the newer atypical antipsychotic medications or the newer antidepressants. The Cubans blame the U.S. embargo for the scarcity of medications. Most medications in Cuba come from Mexico, Venezuela, and other Latin American countries and from Canada and Europe. Although it is likely that the embargo contributes to psychotropic medication shortages, there is also the matter of selectivity. Psychotropic medications are low on the list of those that the government is willing to purchase. Cuba does have a small pharmacological manufacturing industry where some psychotropic medications are produced in limited quantities. For most patients with psychosis, Haldol is used; and for depression, the tricyclic antidepressants, such as Imipramine, are available. These medications are prescribed to people who regularly attend sessions at clinics; of course, many people do not attend. In most cases, the medicines are free or available at very low cost, but sometimes pharmacies run out of supplies and patients have to wait to get their medicines. The Cubans' access to medicines is contrasted with the pharmacies open only to tourists, where most over-the-counter and some prescription medications are available. One Cuban complained that the medicines that Cuba does produce go out to other countries: "It is easier to get Cuban aspirin in Venezuela than in Havana." It is true that exportation of medications and over-the-counter health products does bring income to the Cuban government.

Canada and European countries conduct clinical trials in Cuba's psychiatric facilities. This serves as a way Cuban psychiatrists get the newer medications. Another way is by asking tourists, including those from the United States to bring medications to Cuba. Americans and people from other countries bring medications in on a regular basis, so much so that many clinics count on "tourist drugs." One psychiatrist interviewed stated that she collected as much of one type of medication as possible until she had a six-month supply. That way she could offer it to a patient without the concern that in a few weeks it would run out.

The overall result of having fewer medications to rely upon is the use of talk therapy, mostly cognitive, and other psychosocial interventions. As one psychiatrist reported: "We do therapy because it works. Medications are important, but they are not always the answer. And Cubans don't like to take them, so it works out well for us."

Conclusion

Cubans are notoriously adept at making the most out of limited resources, and their achievements in mental-health treatment are no exception. They subscribe to the concepts of primary and secondary prevention and to using sociological methods to complement traditional psychological and biological treatments. In this way, they overcome the disadvantage of scarce economic resources. Still, Cubans have their own unique problems related to mental health. High suicide rates, alcoholism, poor transportation to clinics, continuing stigma, and limited medications are challenges to their mental-health system.

Perhaps the greatest challenge that mental health professionals face is compiling and reporting on treatment effectiveness. Demographics related to admissions, diagnoses, discharges, and the like are compiled by their Department of Health Systems Statistics and Health Tendencies. There are ongoing efforts to survey a limited number of facilities for outcome data, but currently, national treatment outcome information is not available. Clinical trials are being conducted but on a very limited scale. According to a prominent neuropsychiatrist, data collection to determine the most effective treatments is a priority, and plans are underway for large-scale implementation. There are also no available public data on the treatment of mental illness in diverse groups within Cuba such as the Afro-Cubans and Chinese-Cubans. Cuban health policy does not consider race and ethnic differences as special categories for treatment (World Health Organization, 2005).

When outcome data become available we will know more about the effectiveness of the Cuban system of working with patients with mental illness. Nevertheless, the unique qualities of the Cuban mental-health system are a good fit for a country with limited economic resources and large numbers of mental-health practitioners.

References

Caplan, G. (1964). *The principles of preventive psychiatry.* New York: Basic Books.

Card, D. (1989). The impact of the Mariel BoatLift on the Miami labor market. Working Paper #253, Industrial Relations Section, Princeton University. Retrieved on April 20, 2008, from http://www.irs.princeton.edu/pubs/pdfs/253.pdf

Collinson, S. R., & Turner, T. H. (2002). Not just salsa and cigars: Mental health care in Cuba. *Psychiatric Bulletin, 26,* 185–188.

Donaldson, R. J., & Donaldson, L. J. (1994). *Essential public health medicine.* Lancaster, England: Kluwer.

Greene, R. (2003). Effective community health participation strategies: A Cuban example. *International Journal of Health Planning and Management, 18,* 105–116.

Inter American Commission on Human Rights. (1997). *Report on Cuba.* Retrieved April 20, 2008, from http://www.fiu.edu/~fcf/IACHR.html#IV

Kates, N. (1987). Mental health services in Cuba. *Hospital and Community Psychiatry, 38*(7), 755–758.

McGorry, P. D., & Jackson, H. J. (1999). *The recognition and management of early psychosis.* Cambridge, England: Cambridge University Press.

Medicina Cubana. (2006, 12 August). Cuban doctor imprisoned in psychiatric ward.Retrieved on January 19, 2008, from http://medicinacubana.blogspot.com/2006/08/cuban-doctor-imprisoned-in-psychiatric.htm

Otero-Ojeda, A. A. (2002). *Third Cuban Glossary of Psychiatry (GC-3)*: Key features and contributions. *Psychopathology, 35,* 181–184.

Perez, Jr., L. A. (2005). *To die in Cuba, suicide and society.* Chapel Hill, NC: University of North Carolina Press.

Skaine, R. (2003). *The Cuban family, custom and change.* Jefferson, NC: McFarland.

Spiegel, J. M., González, M., Cabrera, G. J., Catasus, S., Vidal, C., & Yassí, A. (2007, December, 14). (E-publication ahead of print) Promoting health in response to global tourism expansion in Cuba. *Health Promotion International.* Retrieved January 3, 2008, from http://www.liu.xplorex.com/?p2=/modules/liu/publications/view.jsp&id=2074

Vandiver, V. L. (1998). Quality of life, gender and schizophrenia: A cross-national survey in Canada, Cuba, and U.S.A. *Community Mental Health Journal, 34*(6), 501–511.

Warner, R. (2001). The prevention of schizophrenia. What interventions are safe and effective? *Schizophrenia Bulletin, 27*(4), 551–562.

Wasserman, D., Cheng, Q., & Jiang, G. (2005). Global suicide rates among young people aged 15–19. *World Psychiatry, 4*(2), 114–120.

World Health Organization. (2005). *Mental health atlas, 2005.* Retrieved April 20, 2008, from http://www.who.int/mental_health/evidence/atlas/profiles_countries_c_d_.pdf

World Health Organization. (2007). *Mental health.* Retrieved April 20, 2008, from http://www.who.int/mental_health/prevention/suicide/country_reports/en/index.html

CHAPTER SIXTEEN

Psychology in the Community

Jeanne Parr Lemkau

Since my first visit to Cuba, in 2000, when I participated in an educational tour of the Cuban health-care system, I have been a student of psychology on the island, eager to learn about the evolution and practice of my discipline in a sociocultural context so distinct from that of the United States. Between 2000 and 2007, I made seven trips to Cuba with the goal of understanding health care and the role of psychologists, spending more than five months pursuing these interests. I have had the privilege of visiting and informally interviewing several dozen psychologists in various settings in Havana, Santiago de Cuba, and Pinar del Río. My contacts have included psychologists working in universities, polyclinics, mental-health and sports-medicine clinics, residential sanatoria for patients with leprosy and AIDS, a church-related civic organization, hospitals, and a community-based center for HIV/AIDS education and support. In 2001 and 2003, I attended international congresses on women and gender issues organized by an academic psychologist and heavily attended by Cuban psychologists, and the 2003 Congreso Bienal de Psicología en Santiago de Cuba where I presented a day-long work-

I am grateful to the many professionals in Cuba who shared their time, expertise, and example to teach me about psychology in their country.

shop on grief and traumatic loss. On multiple trips, I have spoken at length to several officers of the Society of Cuban Psychologists.

In this chapter, I will summarize what I have learned about the various ways in which psychologists are involved in community work in Cuba. In addition to drawing on knowledge gained from my interchanges in Cuba, I will draw on published literature and on documents graciously provided to me by my Cuban colleagues, including the code of ethics for psychologists, training curricula, and articles in the *Revista Cubana de Psicología*. Where possible, I have attempted to check my understandings with Cuban colleagues. Nevertheless, the conclusions offered here are my own and should be considered with appreciation for the limits of language and cross-cultural research.

Background

Writing in 1985, Bernal described the features of what he saw as a "uniquely Cuban" paradigm of psychology that had evolved from the country's unusual history:

> First, it is a pragmatic, action-oriented model focused on resolving social and community needs in areas such as health and education. Second, as a profession it aims to produce and incorporate research psychologists and other professionals into activities ranging from working with preschoolers and athletes to treating the chronic care patient. Third, while historically influenced by the North American and the Soviet models, this psychology reached beyond both of these to produce a psychology rooted in the contemporary Cuban socio-cultural reality. . . . Lastly, the paradigm is a dialectical one that aims at modifying and impacting the social context. Whereas psychology during the earlier periods can be characterized as applied oriented, during the revolutionary period this orientation flowered into community action and social change. Cuban psychologists today are active in the process of social transformation and participate in moving society toward social and collective ideals. (p. 234)

While more detailed coverage is available elsewhere (Averasturi, 1980; Bernal, 1985; De la Torre & Vales-Fauly, 1996; González Serra, 2003b), I will note some of the historical antecedents that have contributed to the distinctiveness of this Cuban paradigm.

The history of psychology in Cuba is inextricably related to the unique socio-historical conditions of the country (Averasturi, 1980;

González Serra, 2003b). Contemporary psychology in Cuba has been shaped by the legacy of José Martí, the realities of the Cuban revolution, and the influence of Soviet psychology, these factors intermingling with the early and distinctive contributions of Cuban philosophers and psychologists and with the dominant trends of twentieth-century psychology in the United States, Europe, and Latin America.

The nineteenth-century Cuban philosophers Félix Varela Morales and Jose de la Luz y Caballero and the ideals and example of national hero, writer, and poet José Martí set the stage for the later rise of a scientific psychology. Varela's contributions included an exploration of the role of sensory experience in the acquisition of knowledge, a focus on the human capacity for creative thinking, and the pursuit of educational innovation and reform. De la Luz emphasized the importance of subjectivity and the interrelationship between facts and abstraction in creating knowledge and, like Varela, contributed to educational reform (Bernal, 1985). The subsequent scholarship of Enrique José Varona in the early twentieth century established psychology as an empirically based discipline separate from philosophy.

The thinking of Varela and de la Luz y Caballero was formative for José Martí, who was taught by a student of de la Luz (González Serra, 2003a). José Martí saw human personality as a reflection of social reality and saw individual creativity, nurtured through education and example, as determining the course of human development. He emphasized responsibility, self-determination, an orientation to the common good, and the importance of education and example in the development of character and altruism, and personally exemplified the fierce nationalism and self-sacrifice that continue as cultural ideals in Cuba today. Martí emphasized that everyone should study and everyone should teach; hence he has had a strong influence on pedagogical psychology. His influence is also evident (although not explicit) in the current emphasis on community. As expressed by González Serra, the Martían ideal presents a view of humanity and a perspective for a superior society for which Cuban psychology must strive.

Prior to the revolution of 1959, most psychologists in Cuba were trained abroad. Upon their return, they naturally brought to Cuban psychology the dominant theories and paradigms of the United States and Europe, including psychoanalysis, behaviorism, and psychological testing. Psychology was largely practiced within the private sector (Lourdes, 1980), often serving profit-making interests (Averasturi, 1980). There was a strong emphasis on psychometrics, and psychologists usually worked in subordinate positions in relation to psychiatrists.

After *el triunfo de la Revolución,* psychology was infused with Marxist-Leninist ideals and built on the foundation of prerevolutionary psychology and the pervasive influence of José Martí on the national psyche. The first text integrating Marxism with Cuban psychology was published in 1960 (González Martín). Occidental psychotherapies such as psychoanalysis, systems theory, and behaviorism were analyzed from a Marxist-Leninist perspective, with the goal of developing interventions appropriate to Cuban conditions and revolutionary ideology (Averasturi, 1980). The private practice of psychology was eliminated and the scope of practice expanded dramatically as psychologists were recruited to assume new roles in the public-health system and in other public sectors.

The close alliance between Cuba and the Soviet Union in the 1970s and '80s resulted in many Cubans receiving their advanced training in Moscow. As a result, Cuban psychology was also strongly influenced by the work of Russian psychologists, the most important of whom was Lev Vygotsky, whose emphasis on the importance of socio-historical context in determining the course of human development offered a framework consonant with the ideas of José Martí and uniquely suited to the Cuban situation. The major focus of his work was on the crucial role of social interaction in the development of cognition (Vygotsky, 1978). He saw potential cognitive achievement at any given age as limited to a certain range and dependent on social interaction, and proposed the concept of a "zone of proximal development" to refer to the potential that could be attained with optimal social interaction. Accordingly, individual development and achievement could be maximized by adult guidance and peer collaboration.

Consistent with their unique history, Cuban psychologists are taught to view humans as "reflective creators" within socio-historical contexts and to a Marxist-Leninist perspective on social phenomena. Their unusual legacy is evident in a perusal of the *Revista Cubana de Psicología*, where articles on José Martí intermingle with updates on Rorschach testing. Similarly, the standard university curricula for psychology include required courses on the Cuban Revolution and political economics along with the more expected ones on human development and personality assessment.

The fertile mix of historical influences is further evident in conversations with Cuban psychologists. I routinely asked my colleagues the question, "What theorists most influence your work?" Without exception, the first person mentioned by everyone questioned was Vygotsky. Other influential thinkers mentioned included Russian psychologist Lidiya Bozhovich, Carl Rogers, Victor Frankl, and Sigmund Freud, "the behaviorists," and Cubans Varela and Varona. In regard to group work, Paulo Freire (Brazil), Enrique Pichón-Riviere (Argentina), and U.S. sociologist George Homans were also mentioned.

Ethical Guidelines

The character of contemporary psychology in Cuba is reflected in the ethical code of La Sociedad de Psicológos de Cuba, first elaborated in 1989 and revised in 2004. According to the introduction to the more recent version, the mission of the society (the largest and most inclusive of three national organizations that represent psychology, the other two being specifically for health psychologists) is "to construct a scientific community that integrates professionals in both psychology *and related sciences* . . . on behalf of socio-cultural development and human well-being *within the socialist society of Cuba.*" The ethical codes serve "to create and preserve a high level of professionalism which positively influences the contribution of psychology to the solution of problems of human character and *social, economic and other problems of the country.*" Psychologists are expected to "support the development of an *interdisciplinary vision* in research, teaching, and practice." One of the goals of research is to contribute to "*transformations toward perfection of the society of our country.*" (All translations and italics by the author.) These statements illustrate three aspects of psychology in Cuba that are exemplified in community practice: (1) a tendency to work closely and respectfully with "related sciences," (2) a very broad and ambitious scope of practice, and (3) a conception of the field as serving the common good within a socialist society.

The fact that the practice of psychologists integrates both civic values and professional ethics is demonstrated in a study of applied ethics in Cuba, conducted by the Canadian team of Valdés et al. (2002). They conducted in-depth interviews and focus groups with twenty-eight mental-health professionals, including twenty-three psychologists, and concluded that ethics were perceived as central to professional practice, with "a synergy between the professional ideals of service to the community and the revolutionary goals of prosperity for all" (p. 231). Using a grounded theory methodology, they identified a cluster of civic values that informed the work of psychologists, including solidarity, humanism, dignity, and pride in their *Cubanía,* independence from foreign domination, and the promotion of socialism. These professionals revered national poet José Martí for his personification of these values and saw their work as rooted in their history and serving the goals of the revolution to create a more humanitarian society. In discussing the ethical principles that guide their professional practice, respondents included collectivism and community participation along with respect, empathy, and commitment, as well as authenticity, self-respect, and scientific rigor.

In contrast with North American psychologists, Cubans tended to endorse the precept that the personal is political, favor collectivism over individualism, and conceptualize personal difficulties in the context of social problems. One with the valued "revolutionary consciousness" would see individual behavior in terms of the extent to which it benefits the larger society (Lowenthal, Danson, & Lowenthal, 1985, p. 107). González Serra, writing from a Marxist-Leninist perspective and inspired by José Martí, writes that the "superior human being" that psychology should work to foster is characterized by altruism rather than egotism (2003a). He writes:

> Altruism consists in putting in first place the interests of humanity as a whole and especially the requirements of countries and social classes most in need and the most urgent global problems; in second place the interests of the geographical region and the country of one's birth (patriotism); in the third place the necessities of our provinces and zone of residence, in second to last place the family and last, our personal interests. (p. 3)

The importance of both professionals and other citizens in working within their communities and social networks for the collective good is a natural corollary of this perspective. As expressed by Lowenthal and colleagues, "A prime characteristic of Cuban society is to change the very nature of the relationships between people and their social institutions" (1985, p. 113).

Training

There are currently three avenues for becoming a psychologist: through traditional university training, through the *municipalizacion* training in the community (described below), and, for health psychologists, through training by the Ministry of Public Health (MINSAP) in hospital and community settings.

Education to earn the *Licenciatura* takes five years at the university or six through the municipalization program. This level of training, roughly equivalent to the master's degree in the United States, prepares students as generalists for work in a wide variety of settings. This degree, plus one or two years of supervised social service, is required to secure a position as a psychologist. Most psychologists in Cuba are trained at this level. Specialized training at the master's and doctoral degree levels is available through the universities and through MINSAP (for health psychologists), with the highest degree generally pursued only by those intending to enter university teaching or research careers.

The first training program in psychology began at the University of Villanueva in 1952 (Bernal, 1985). Both the University of Havana and the University of Santa Clara began training programs in psychology in 1962.

Beginning in 2002 in Havana and 2003 in most other provinces, it has been possible for students to become psychologists through education provided in community settings, with curricula equivalent to that offered in university settings but spread over six years instead of five. Psychologists educated through this avenue are beginning to complete their social service obligations and swell the workforce of available professionals in the field.

Psychology is highly valued as a profession. "A spirit of collaboration" exists between psychologists and members of other helping professions. Although medical doctors have a higher salary and higher status, no one has real economic privilege, a fact that may contribute to the ease of collaboration. One psychologist reported that he felt a "*gran hermanidad*" [great brotherhood] with his medical colleagues when they worked side by side in a polyclinic.

Psychologists' Roles in the Community

Psychologists serve their communities in a myriad of ways, since they are employed in virtually every sector of Cuban society—from education to government to industry to health care. Some roles and situations in which psychologists serve their communities are described below. This list is not exhaustive.

POPULAR EDUCATION

Psychologists are involved in designing, coordinating, and executing popular education initiatives in various settings, following the methodology of Brazilian Paulo Freire (1999) to encourage individuals to become informed and active in addressing social issues. The Martin Luther King Center (MLK) in Havana (Marianao), one of the strongest nongovernmental organizations in Cuba, is an ecumenical religious organization devoted to fostering progressive change in Cuba and Latin America, and the major force for popular education in Cuba.

The King Center has a staff of about forty people, half of whom are involved in program coordination. Since the 1980s, psychologists on the MLK staff have designed and executed training workshops for community and church leaders using popular education methods. Through these programs, psychologists promote social involvement and leadership development in such different arenas as the environment, gender, agriculture, and Christian education. When asked to describe typical responsibilities of her position, a psychologist who coordinates popular education at MLK mentioned preparing distance-learning modules in popular education, evaluating the effectiveness of current programs, preparing new courses, writing articles, and studying to keep up with new approaches to community work.

Psychologists are also involved in popular education elsewhere, for example in settings devoted to AIDS prevention and/or to the support of patients who are HIV positive or have AIDS. At the AIDS Sanatorium at Santiago de Las Vegas, popular education informs the work of psychologists with groups.

"MUNICIPALIZATION"

Several years ago, Cuba initiated a program nationwide to bring university training opportunities to the community through evening classes available to all. Psychologists have been crucial to the success of this "municipalization" initiative. As the opportunity to pursue university education and training for the field of psychology spread into the community, the need for psychologists as teachers dramatically increased. Since one can also pursue other social science careers through this program (including communication, history, law, library and information science, and social-cultural studies) and psychology courses are required by all students as part of a common first-year curriculum, psychologists have a critical role in the success of this nationwide educational innovation. Although they are not required to do so, many psychologists teach in the evenings in addition to their day jobs in other settings, receiving a small stipend for doing so.

Classes typically meet for two hours every two weeks, with study and assignments in the community between classes. Books are provided to students on a loan basis. Students also have tutorial groups and meet with their tutors regularly, about once a month, and many of these tutors are psychologists. The purpose of tutorial groups is to encourage and support the work that students do in their classes and required practicum experiences. On-the-job training is integrated into the curriculum, and the relationship between the program and other community institutions is two-way, with many students pursuing schooling at the recommendations of community leaders.

I was able to meet with a group of four mental-health professionals who teach psychology and an advanced psychology student in the municipalization program in Central Havana. During the day, these psychologists were variously employed in a sports-medicine clinic, a mental-health center, and a polyclinic. The fourth was on medical disability from her long-term employment, but still chose to participate in evening teaching. Although they knew each other from regular meetings of their teaching cluster devoted to reviewing both curricular content and teaching methodology, until it came up in discussion, the fact that one woman was not a psychologist but a psychiatrist was not known by the others. I was told, in this and other settings, that one's discipline was not as important as the work that one does and the sense of team and mission with the group. I was also assured that only psychologists supervise those who teach psychology courses.

The curriculum for training psychologists is fixed with limited elective possibilities. It is the equivalent to that offered in the traditional university setting, although there is more emphasis on self-study and on finding resources in the community to enhance the classroom experience. For example, students taking a course on human development were instructed to find a place in their neighborhood where they could observe and study children of different ages. Faculty members are approved through the regular university, and required exams are the same in both systems.

Prior to the municipalization program, only those who qualified through specific tests were allowed to enter the field of psychology. With this program, the field has opened up to all who are able to complete their studies and pass the required exams. One psychologist voiced the opinion that with teaching in the community, psychologists have become more oriented to social problems and less focused on those of individuals.

The student present was in her fifth year. Her current practicum was in group therapy in Old Havana. She had completed other practicum experiences at the AIDS sanatorium and on an organ transplant unit of the major international hospital. As a student she had been allowed to attend several scientific congresses and international meetings held in Cuba and related to her interests.

The group of psychologist/teachers with whom I met was notable for their enthusiasm and sense of shared purpose. One woman explained that she volunteers to teach because she finds it a very satisfying way to contribute to her community. "Ours is a poor neighborhood, and even if our students don't always graduate, at least while they are with us they aren't in the streets." She saw her role as one of encouragement and support and was moved when someone on the street called her "*Mi profi*."

While the municipalization program exemplifies integration of psychologists into the community, the work of academic psychologists in traditional university settings often extends into the community as well, via research, provision of care, and coordination/monitoring of municipalization teachers.

Community Mental Health

There is no private consultation in psychology in Cuba. It is against professional ethics and against the law (González Sierra, November 28, 2007, personal communication). All psychologists are employed by the state. Most psychologists devoted to mental health work in polyclinics and mental-health centers. Their integration into the public-health system and primary-care medicine began in the mid-1960s and has been given high priority for many years. Psychologists in polyclinics typically work within multidisciplinary teams, and have been vitally involved in educational activities, psychotherapy, and intervention in the community milieu for several decades (Averasturi, 1980; Félix Sanso, personal communication, 2003).

There are more than four hundred polyclinics in the country, serving about fifteen thousand neighborhood *consultorios,* where doctor-nurse teams attend to the primary-care needs of a defined group of families (vice minister of MINSAP for international affairs, personal communication, January 2005). These teams may consult with or refer to the psychologist at the polyclinic in regard to the mental-health needs of their patients. Individuals may also self-refer to these psychologists or to mental-health professionals at mental-health centers.

The community mental-health center is very involved in serving the needs of its municipality with such activities as parenting classes, support for caretakers, group treatment for alcoholics, and so on. Psychologists are involved in all of these activities. These centers sometimes initiate "neighborhood debates," educational and interactive programs where psychologists and others lead discussions about community problems and how they might be addressed.

The community mental-health centers are both multidisciplinary and interdisciplinary, and psychologists there help individuals and families link with other organizations such as health centers, the Federation of Cuban Women, and the municipalization programs. A psychologist employed at a mental-health center mentioned that he frequently referred patients to the municipalization program as a way to go back to school and better their situation. He found it especially satisfying when individuals who had been imprisoned were able to become educated.

PHYSICAL HEALTH

Cuba boasts the lowest rate of HIV/AIDS in the Caribbean, and many psychologists are involved in the prevention of AIDS and in the treatment and support of HIV-positive and AIDS patients. Psychologists at the regional center for AIDS prevention in Pinar del Río described their roles in this regard.

At the center, a psychologist who answers questions and encourages anonymous testing for HIV/AIDS (a service provided by the center and not available through the polyclinics) works with an epidemiologist to analyze AIDS-related problems in the community. Another psychologist working to address such problems had shown a popular Cuban movie, *Lucía,* to a group of women from the community, using the film to stimulate discussion about aspects of women's behavior such as gender roles, and violence against women that contributed to high-risk behavior. A third psychologist provided psychotherapy support to people who were HIV-positive or had AIDS.

One psychologist had worked at a nearby residential detention center where women served several years for prostitution and other crimes. She began her work with the intention of training the women to become health promoters in their communities upon discharge, but in the process of getting to know them discovered problems of self-esteem, deficient social skills, and need for reeducation in regard to basic values. She continued working with the women on the problems she identified. She says that her experience has taught her that it is "important to hold both social and clinical perspectives at the same time." The same psychologist also contributed to a weekly radio show that includes psychological content related to AIDS prevention, along with musical programming.

Psychologists who work at the center have organized meetings with representatives of the Federation of Cuban Women and faculty working on family curricula at the University of Pinar del Río to identify possible linkages. One of them had taught a class at the university the day before that had focused on AIDS. Psychologists were also involved in evaluating community programs through observation and interviews. One psychologist described the process as, "first qualitative diagnosis, then intervention and evaluation."

Many of the psychologists who work in AIDS prevention work in other areas as well. For example, one psychologist who had been trained at MLK in popular education, uses this methodology in classes with medical students focusing on environmental factors related to health and with community groups working toward sustainable development.

The majority of psychologists work in primary care through the polyclinics, under the rubric of MINSAP. Psychologists are involved in the prevention of illness through education and in treatment and palliative care. Some teach in the medical schools. The involvement of psychologists in the physical-health arena includes programmatic development, teaching, direct service, media, and research. The variety of their responsibilities suggests an unusually broad scope of practice, with an emphasis on social and collective factors. For example, first-year students in health psychology have been asked to participate in anti-dengue campaigns by visiting people in their homes and encouraging them to clean up standing water that breeds mosquitoes.

MEDIA

Psychologists are integrated into a variety of radio and TV programs throughout the country and contribute to printed media for the public.

The daily TV show, *Universidad para Todos* [University for Everyone] often includes psychological content. Psychologists from the University of Havana initiated a popular radio show called *Vale la Pena* [It's Worth It] that includes advice and presentations by psychologists. They also contribute to a weekly newspaper for workers called *Trajabadores*.

The contributions of psychologists through the media often interrelate with their other roles. A psychologist in Pinar del Río recalled hosting a radio show in which a man called in and argued for a half hour trying to defend what the psychologist saw as physical abuse of his son. On the show, she did her best to give him another perspective. Shortly thereafter, a woman approached her on the street of her community and said, "That was my husband," and the psychologist was able to begin a dialogue with the family.

OTHER SETTINGS WHERE PSYCHOLOGISTS ARE INVOLVED WITH THE COMMUNITY

Psychologists are involved in community-oriented research—often interdisciplinary in nature—as part of their responsibilities in health and social service settings, through universities, and within MINSAP and other ministries of the government. The most important social research in the country is conducted by the Center for Investigations in Psychology and Sociology (CIPS), an interdisciplinary center under the Ministry for Science, Technology, and Environment. It was founded by a social psychologist who directed the center for many years and also served as vice minister of the ministry.

In the work sector, psychologists are involved in evaluating and promoting job satisfaction and promotion and in the selection of workers. Some are employed to work in the tourism sector, of crucial importance to the economy of Cuba. Their roles include promoting tourism and training tour guides in human relations.

Psychologists have been involved in innovative programs for the elderly. For example, psychologists at the University of Havana originated a community-education program for elders, La Universidad de La Tercera Edad, which was expanded nationwide. In informal group settings, this program educates older people on topics related to health, nutrition, and daily living.

Conclusions

The descriptions I have offered are based on a small sampling of psychologists and settings in a country with eleven million people, shaped by my North American perspective and imperfect understanding. My interchanges with Cuban psychologists have not included opportunities for directly observing them in their work roles and settings. What does thinking in "socio-historical context" look like in practice? How does thinking of people as "reflective creators" shape interventions? How do Cuban psychologists behave differently from their counterparts elsewhere? A more in-depth understanding would require both observation and research at the micro-level on how their psychological perspectives are translated into practice, and on how the contributions of psychologists differ and/or overlap with those of other professionals.

Psychological education and training is relevant to any job that involves human relations, and Cuban psychologists have demonstrated their worth, flexibility, and skills in a plethora of settings. Nevertheless, the increasing breadth of the field may bring problems for the discipline. In a country where psychologists work everywhere and where interdisciplinary and multidisciplinary work is the norm, distinctions between fields may blur and the relationship between psychological practice and the science of psychology may stretch to the breaking point. As one young psychologist put it, "Psychology used to be an elite field. Now psychologists are doing everything and I wonder whether we will lose our identity." At the same time, because the pragmatic orientation and mixing of professions provides such fertile ground for innovation, and hypothesis generation and testing, the evolution and content of psychology in Cuba compels the interest of an international audience.

In Cuba, as in other countries, psychology is a social *science*, and as such, dependent on the continual interplay of evaluation and experimentation. Regrettably, material resources to support scientific investigation are in short supply in Cuba owing to the economic situation on the island, made worse by the U.S. embargo. The professional journals, books, psychometric instruments, computers, and other materials needed to conduct research are scarce (Sleek, 1999). Internet access and opportunities for travel abroad are limited, crippling interchange with the international community of psychologists. These factors constrain the extent to which Cubans can empirically evaluate their programs and contribute to the advancement of psychology as a science. This is unfortunate for Cuba and for the discipline of psychology, since more scientific evaluation of the work of Cuban psychologists in the community could offer unique contributions to our understanding of what works in what contexts and why.

In my interactions with Cuban psychologists over the past eight years, I have been impressed with their warmth, energy, sincerity, and commitment—to their profession, their country, and to the goals of socialism. Their devotion to applying their professional skills for the collective good is inspiring. Cuban psychologists are involved in virtually every sector of the Cuban workforce, impacting their communities in a broad array of multidisciplinary and interdisciplinary settings. As increasing numbers of psychologists graduate from the innovative municipalization training program, the involvement of psychologists in various aspects of community work can be expected to expand even further. Their orientation to work on behalf of the common good offers a needed counterpoint to the dominant paradigm of the United States that places primacy on individual well-being.

References

Averasturi, L. G. (1980). Psychology and health care in Cuba. *American Psychologist, 35*(12), 1090–1095.

Bernal G. (1985). History of psychology in Cuba. *Journal of Community Psychology, 13*(2), 222–235.

Código de Ética de la Sociedad de Psicologos de Cuba.(2004). (Full citation and pagination not available; provided through personal communication with officer of Society of Cuban Psychologists).

De la Torre, M. C., & Vales-Fauly, M. V. (1996). Logros, problemas y retos de la psicología en Cuba. *Revista Cubana de Psicología, 13*(2–3).

Freire, P. (1999). *Pedagogy of the oppressed.* New York: Continuum Publishing.

González Martin, D. (1960). Experimentos e Ideología. Bases de una teoría psicológica. Merida, Mexico: Universidad de los Andes.

González Serra, D. J. (2003a). La psicología ye el futuro de la humanidad. *Revista Cubana de Psicología*, Supplement 1.-

González Serra, D. J. (2003b). *La psicología en Cuba: Actualidad y perspectivas.* Paper presented at the 2003 Congreso bienal de psicología in Santiago de Cuba.

Lourdes, A. (1980). Psychology and health care in Cuba. *American Psychologist, 35*(12), 1090–1095.

Lowenthal A. S., Danson C., & Lowenthal, B. B. (1985, April). Psychology and human services in Cuba: Personal perspectives. *Journal of Community Psychology, 13*(2), 105–116.

Sleek, S. (1999, February). In Cuba, a revolution bypasses psychology. *Monitor on Psychology, 30*(2), Retrieved February 5, 2008, from http://www.apa.org/monitor/feb99/cuba.html

Valdés, L. S., Prilleltensky, I., Walsh-Bowers, R., & Rossiter, A. (2002). Applied ethics on mental health in Cuba, part 1. *Ethics and Behavior, 12*(3), 223–242.

Vygotsky, L. S. (1978). *Mind in society: The development of higher psychological processes.* Cambridge, MA: Harvard University Press.

CHAPTER SEVENTEEN

Music Therapy in Cuba

Melanie Nevis

Music in Cuba is everywhere—in the streets, in restaurants, in backyard rumbas, in every home, in cultural gatherings and religious ceremonies. It is an integral part of life in Cuba and a crucial aspect of Cuban cultural identity and pride. While music traditions are revered, Cuban music continues to develop in the *calle* [street] and is continually growing and creating new forms and traditions. Cuba does not manifest the same degree of "functional integration" (Chernoff, 1979, p. 33) between music and culture as seen in African traditions, where virtually every community event has musical rituals to express it. Nevertheless, aspects of these traditions continue in Cuba, and Cuban folkloric music is a strong part of spiritual, cultural, and emotional expression. Cuba is acknowledged as having world-class music conservatories and classical music training, placing strong emphasis on and taking great pride in the high quality of its musicians. At the same time, Cuba has embraced alternative approaches in community health with its internationally recognized Western medical training and care.

How does music's use as a therapeutic modality in community health care fit with the overall model of health care in Cuba? This chapter explores this question, focusing on three areas of inquiry: (1) the cultural and historical use of music as a therapeutic or healing modality in

Cuban culture, (2) current developments in music therapy in Cuba, and (3) the intercultural collaboration with mental-health communities in Cuba.

Cuban Folkloric Music: A Cultural/Historical Perspective

"Music is so essential to the Cuban character that you can't disentangle it from the history of the nation. The history of Cuban music is one of cultural collisions, of voluntary and forced migrations, of religions and revolution." (Ned Sublette, Cuba and Its Music).

In addressing music therapy in community health care in Cuba, it is important to understand and acknowledge the impact of Cuba's cultural and folkloric music traditions. Cuban music evolved from the confluence of three cultures: African, Spanish, and Indian, although the primary influences came from Spain and Africa. When Spain colonized Cuba in the early 1500s, it enslaved and then eliminated two to three million indigenous Cuban Indians, including the inhabitants of Taino, Sibony, and Guanajatabibe, as well as other Caribe tribes. These groups exerted less influence over Cuban music because the European Jesuit missionaries, in their zeal to convert the Indians to Christianity, suppressed the Indians' cultural practices. However, it is believed that the use of shakers and rattles evolved from the indigenous Indian peoples (Uribe, 1996).

By the sixteenth century, the Spanish had virtually eliminated the Indians and their cultural influence. Dissatisfied with the work of the Indian slaves, the Spanish had begun to bring in African slaves to work the lucrative Cuban sugar crop (Uribe, 1996). The majority of the slaves were from the Yoruban culture of West Africa, but slaves with the sacred and secular drumming traditions of the Abakuá, Dahomean, and Congolese cultures also were brought to Cuba.

These African slaves brought with them highly developed vocal and rhythmic elements, and they began to re-create their drums and other percussion instruments (Uribe, 1996). While the music that developed was distinctly Cuban, many of the cultural, rhythmic, and spiritual aspects of African drumming traditions became an integral part of Cuban folkloric music. Many elements of the music and dance of these African people are clearly seen in the secular folkloric and religious music of Cuba.

The Spanish sought to suppress the religious and musical culture of the Africans, forcing them to learn Spanish as their primary language and practice Christianity in the form of Catholicism. Seeking to hide their native African religious and magical practices from the Spaniards, African slaves in Cuba identified their deities with the Catholic saints (González-Whippler, 1996). In this way, they held on to their traditional values, beliefs, and musical elements, and "among themselves, they worshipped the saints with the songs and dances of their motherland" (Murphy, 1988, p. 2). This activity resulted in syncretism, "the spontaneous, popular combination or reconciliation of different religious beliefs" (González-Whippler, 1996, p. 3); in Cuba these practices became known as Lucumí, or Santería—a worship of the saints. Santería's worship rituals and ceremonies involve extensive drumming and singing, and to this day retain many traditional musical characteristics of African Yoruban singing and drumming.

Cuban folkloric music is not traditionally viewed as being used specifically for healing purposes, although there are anecdotal reports of its healing effects (Nevis, 2001). Cuban folkloric music is viewed as an integral part of the culture, with much therapeutic, religious, spiritual, social, emotional, and artistic importance. Within Cuban folkloric music, two distinct genres can be identified. The first, mentioned briefly above, consists of the religious music of Santería and other African-derived religions, while the second genre comprises the secular folkloric music of Cuba (such as rumba or *comparsa*). The environment, purpose, and meaning of the secular and religious types of folkloric music are different, but both consist of important interactions between the musicians and community participants, and both retain many important elements of African musical and cultural influences.

Sacred Folkloric Music—Santería

In the religious Santería ceremony, the purpose of the music is to summon the orisha (saint) for trance possession. The possessed person, embodying the orisha, can then give counsel and spiritual advice to those gathered at the ceremonies. The specific rhythms, songs, and dances of Santería combine to call the orisha and to "entrance" the participant, so that he or she is open and susceptible to possession. Santería ceremonies generally take place in the homes of initiates or priests of the religion. The central purpose of the ritual itself is to honor the orishas, and the ceremonies are held for various reasons: to initiate people into the religion of Santería, to celebrate the sacred day of an orisha, to celebrate the anniversary of a person's initiation into Santería, to honor an elder in the religion, or to express gratitude or tribute to an orisha. Santería ceremonies are also used to ask for help or assistance, often regarding health and personal problems.

Secular Folkloric Music: Rumba

Among the most prominent secular folkloric music traditions in Cuba is the culture of rumba, "a secular dance/music/poetic expression that developed among the various African ethnic groups first brought to Cuba" (Crook, 1992, p. 31). Rumba is traditionally performed with percussion, vocals, and dancers. It draws its primary influences from the Bantú Congolese people and the folkloric Spanish song styles of flamenco and rumba flamenco, but it has been influenced by other religious and secular African folkloric styles as well. It originated among nineteenth-century groups known as *córos de clave*, which performed in the streets and neighborhoods in Cuba. Rumba remains a part of neighborhood and community culture. It is much more than a rhythm: it is a fiesta, a gathering, and a musical and dance style with its own cultural and musical language. Rumba uses call and response, and depends on the interactions between singers, dancers, drummers, and the gathered community. Participants take turns drumming, singing, and dancing, with each contributor competing to outshine the one who came before.

Therapeutic Effects of Cuban Folkloric Music: Current Research Findings

In 2000, I completed a research study in Cuba entitled "The Therapeutic Aspects of Cuban Folkloric Drumming." Under the guidance of a renowned percussionist and the Cuban organization PERCUBA, I interviewed and videotaped twenty-five musicians ranging from renowned self-taught folkloric masters to highly educated musicians/musicologists. As one of the few nongovernmental music organizations in Cuba, PERCUBA is a group of professional percussionists and musicologists who, among other activities, produce a yearly conference and festival of folkloric and contemporary percussion. The project consisted of interviews, surveys, videos, observations, and attendances at folkloric music fiestas and ceremonies. This study addressed the effects of specific rhythms, the personal experiences of drummers and listeners, the impact of the environment and culture where drumming occurs, drumming-induced trance and altered states, and the comparative effects of listening and playing. My goal was to use this knowledge to integrate the therapeutic effects of traditional drumming into the clinical requirements of the music-therapy field.

All the musicians and musicologists interviewed believed that drumming and folkloric music have therapeutic effects on both player and listener. They reported that these effects result in a shift of energy, emotion, and physical sensations. The drumming and folkloric music produced relaxation, stress reduction, excitement, motivation, increased energy, and decreased depression and anxiety. Also reported were a decrease in physical symptoms and pain, euphoria, happiness, and a change in psychosomatic symptoms. Although it is not considered folkloric music's primary purpose, many musicians believed that they had been personally healed with drumming and folkloric music; others gave specific examples of people, including family members, being healed of illnesses from listening to folkloric music, even in nonreligious settings. All the musicians interviewed stressed that music is an important expression of their emotions. They also identified some specific effects of certain rhythms on themselves as follows: "If I have pain or illness, it is gone, I don't feel it"; "It's like a meditation, it calms me"; "It energizes and motivates me"; "I forget all my problems and struggles"; "I am happy"; "I leave myself—I can go to another place."

Cuban folkloric musicians also spoke of the importance and profound impact of playing together in a community gathering—the energy exchange, the communication, the sense of being an important part of a polyrhythmic whole that is greater than the individual—were all uniquely important experiences for them. Many of the people interviewed stressed the therapeutic effects on the listener as well as the musician. It is important to understand that the concept of "listening" to music is not passive in an African or Cuban setting; to listen to music in a Cuban folkloric setting is to be an active participant. The music and drumming are one aspect of the larger social/communal/religious gathering of drummers, singers, and dancers. If you are listening, you are probably also moving, dancing, and singing along with the chorus. The energy and improvisations of the drummers feed directly off the dancers and singers—and vice versa—so that every participant is involved in the conversation and creation of the music in a larger sense. Dancing and singing contribute to the strong rhythmic entrainment that occurs, and to the social and emotional sense of being part of the whole.

Rumba

The therapeutic effects of rumba and other nonreligious music at fiestas and gatherings are viewed by most musicians primarily as stress reducers. Forgetting your problems, expressing yourself, improvising and creating through singing, dancing, playing instruments, bring both musicians and listeners into a group or community and contribute to a reduction of stress. The emphasis on communication between the drummers, singers, and dancers in the community gathering plays a crucial part in the therapeutic effects of the music.

Santería Music

In Cuba, the impact of Santería on the culture is deep and widespread; even those who are not active practitioners possess significant knowledge about the symbols, beliefs, and music of the religion, often integrating some aspects of Santería into their own beliefs and lives. It is important to be aware of the many influences of Santería's religious and musical aspects on health care and music therapy in Cuba. In discussing the importance of cultural context, Argentinean music therapist Diego Schapira explains: "Let's get back to the sound of the drums. Their sound will evoke different things to someone from Johannesburg, Montevideo, Berlin, or Tokyo" (Schapira, 2002, p. xx). An understanding of the impact and meaning of trance within Santería music, and sensitivity toward the significance of personal and cultural belief systems, are both necessary factors in developing music therapy in community health care in Cuba. In a Santería ceremony, specific rhythms are played to communicate with and to summon specific orishas. Along with the drumming and rhythm, a number of important factors play a part in trance and altered states. The music produces what is known in music therapy as rhythmic entrancement, rhythmically repetitive music, and musical stimuli that affects both physiological and psychological states, an important aspect to consider when examining drumming, trance, and altered states.

It is especially important to understand how music can contribute to or cause a trance or altered state when using Cuban folkloric music or rhythms in a therapy setting. What is often unclear is whether one can separate the impact of ritual and belief from the experience of music, and thus determine how specific musical elements may have psycho-physical effects on a person apart from other meanings. Participants in the study shared numerous examples of musicians or teachers in academic settings going into trance at inappropriate times—when it was neither their desire nor their goal (Nevis, 2001). They also gave specific examples of witnessing bystanders who were not religious, or even focused on the ceremonies, going into trance from the rhythm itself. The issue of going into trance "out of context" raises questions about the strength of the stimuli from the music and drumming itself, and is important to consider in the application of Cuban music in music therapy.

Evolution of the Music-Therapy Field in Cuba

HISTORY OF MUSIC THERAPY IN MEDICINE AND HEALTH CARE

Musicologist Alfredo Hildago-Gato Esquerré has researched the documented history of music therapy in medicine and community health prior to the 2003 formation of a formal Cuban music-therapy association. His research documents the independent development and use of therapeutic music in medicine in Cuba (Hidalgo-Gato Esquerré, personal communication, November 29, 2007).

As early as 1899, Dr. Gordon y de Costa wrote an essay describing his work that examined the effect of music on the body, particularly as it relates to the nervous system. From 1953 to 1955, psychiatrist Diana Laura Rodriquez used music in her treatment of tuberculosis patients in a psychiatric ward and presented the results of her research in 1963 at the X Congreso Médico Nacional at the Hospital Psiquiátrico de La Habana. Gynecologist Celestino Alvarez Lajonchere used music to relax patients during childbirth.

In the 1960s, Dr. Jose Gali García Hernandez also used music in his work with psychiatric patients at a day-treatment program at Hospital Calixto García de La Habana. His program included a collaboration with two renowned Cuban musicians, baritone Ramon Calzadilla and composer Silvio Rodríguez. The early '60s also marked the beginning of the integration of music as a therapeutic mode at the Hospital Psiquiátrico de La Habana by Dr. Gilbertina Puertas. She created a method of therapeutic music that began with passive listening and then developed into more active music making and participation (Puertas, 1975). Further developments in therapeutic music research emerged between the late 1960s and the early 1970s. Dr. Armando Chang at the Hospital Psiquiátrico in Camagüey, and Dr. Armando Córdova and psychologist Elena Iglesias at the Piti Fajardo Hospital, also used music in their treatments. In 1991, concurrent with but separate from the development of the Cuban Music Therapy Association, Lidia Suarte, a music teacher, developed a program of music treatment at La Casteana, a shelter for children and adolescents with physical, health, and developmental disabilities (Fernández de Juan, personal communication, November 29, 2007). All reported positive outcomes resulting from their programs.

While the above represent the documented uses of therapeutic music in Cuba, anecdotal reports also exist (Nevis, 2001). A musician recalled hearing of a physician in the 1970s who had brought folkloric percussionists into a psychiatric hospital for therapeutic purposes. Another person had heard of music being used in a pain clinic. One musician mentioned that he was aware of some psychiatrists who were also *babalawos,* priests in the Santería religion, who had integrated some of the music from Santería in their work.

The Cuban Music Therapy Group

In the 1980s, no training programs or academic studies in music therapy were yet available in Cuba. The creation of the music-therapy field there came through the dedication of a small number of doctors, psychologists, musicians, musicologists, and other health workers. While independently developing their own work, these professionals sought collaboration, teaching, and supervision from music therapists in other countries, primarily Argentina, Brazil, and Spain (Fernández de Juan, personal communication, November 29, 2007). Leading this effort was Cuban music therapist, Dr. Teresa Fernández de Juan, who is the director of the Cuban Music Therapy Group and a researcher at El Colegio de la Frontera Norte, in Tijuana, Mexico. With supervision from Dr. Rolando Benenzon of Argentina, Fernández trained at various centers in Buenos Aires, Argentina, and completed a doctoral program at the Río De Janeiro Music Conservatory in Brazil.

In 1988, the "Training Group of Cuban Music Therapy" began to meet. An informal group, it consisted of various professionals interested in music therapy. This group collaborated with a variety of specialists, including social workers, musicians, musicologists, neurophysiologists, and psychologists, to form the Music Therapy Laboratory of the Academy of Sciences' Centre of Fundamental Brain Investigations. Along with Fernández, a distingushed group of professionals that included neurophysiologists, neuropsychologists, psychologists, social workers, psychiatrists, and musicologists focused their research on the connection between music and neurology. Working together, they did multiple research studies on the diverse therapeutic uses of music (Fernández de Juan, 2003).

At the same time, others in Cuba were conducting research on music's effect on physical conditions, including a study addressing hypertension. One such project, initiated by Dr. Dionisio F. Zaldívar Pérez and Lic. Eridel Peraza Chil showed music to therapeutically lower stress factors in patients with high blood pressure by decreasing anxiety and depression (Peraza Chil & Zaldívar Pérez, 2003). Others, including Dr. Máximo Hernández, of the International School of Cinema and Television of San Antonio de los Baños also began developing alternative therapeutic approaches that included music and sound therapies (Fernández de Juan, 2003).

After joining the Federation of Latin American Music Therapists, Fernández represented the Cuban Association of Music Therapy at World Federation meetings. As this group continued to develop their work, the desire and need to create a scientifically based and internationally recognized music-therapy training program in Cuba grew stronger.

Master's Degree Program in Cuba

In 2007, the Cuban Music Therapy Group announced the formation of the first master's degree program in music therapy in Cuba, chaired by Fernández with support from Diego Schapira, a music therapy professor in Argentina. This program represents a unique collaboration between a music conservatory, the Instituto Superior de Arte, and the psychology department of the University of Havana. The program is to be taught with the support of music therapists from Brazil, Argentina, Spain, Mexico, and the United States, along with Cuban psychologists and musicians. In addition to being Cuba's first music-therapy training program, it will also be the first master's degree program in the Central American and Caribbean region.

At this juncture, the goal of the Cuban Music Therapy Group is twofold: (1) to create a formal academic training program with international standards and requirements and, (2) to support and be inclusive of the independent work and creativity occurring in the country (Fernández de Juan, personal communication, November 29, 2007). Their goals are meant to encourage interested individuals to train formally in music therapy and to develop a means of formal supervision for other professionals who are working with music therapeutically without music therapy degrees. They aim to create a clear understanding of music therapy as an academic and scientific field (Fernández de Juan, personal communication, November 29, 2007). These multiple goals and the challenges that they present are similar to the growing pains experienced by academic and scientific communities in other countries looking to develop a new field and meet international standards. What stands out in the Cuban Music Therapy Group's perspective is its desire and commitment to be as inclusive as possible and to support therapeutic work at the community level.

Integration of Music Therapy in the Community Health-Care System in Cuba

Many professionals at mental health centers, schools, and hospitals in Cuba have independently developed music therapy or therapeutic music programs in community health care. Fernández and the Cuban Music Therapy Group have created several programs and research projects in diverse settings. Two outstanding examples of community music-therapy programs include those at El Centro Comunitario de Salud Mental de Regla and Hospital Psiquiátrico de La Habana, Havana.

El Centro Comunitario de Salud Mental de Regla

Directed by Dr. Raúl Gil Sánchez, the *centro* is an innovative and highly regarded community health center in Regla, a city across the bay from Havana. Renowned as a model community mental-health program both internationally and in Cuba, Dr. Gil and the *centro* have played a large role in the development and legitimization of the therapeutic use of the arts in Cuba. By addressing both the cultural and mental-health needs of the whole community, Dr. Gil has created a center that is truly inclusive of the full community and minimizes the stigma of mental-health treatment. In addition to other alternative health methods, the *centro* has supported the use of music as an integral aspect of community health care and included therapeutic music sessions for both children and seniors. In 2003 and again in 2005, the *centro* sponsored an Arts in Therapy Congress as part of an international mental-health conference in Regla. This event was followed in 2007 with the Bienal de Las Artes y Salud Mental, an arts-in-therapy conference that was included in the month-long international art show, the Habana Bienal, in Havana.

Under the guidance of Fernández, two studies emerged from the Cuban Music Therapy Group, both with roots at the El Centro Comunitario de Salud Mental de Regla.

GERIATRIC MENTAL HEALTH AND MUSIC THERAPY

Beginning in 1998, Dr. Rigoberto Oliva Sánchez, a physician and musician, worked in groups with the elderly at the *centro*. These groups focused on issues of depression, mood disorders, and communication disorders. Between 1998 and 2006, his team completed a series of research studies of geriatric patients who engaged in music-therapy activities. There, earlier studies included having groups participating in music listening, music improvisation, and relaxation techniques to address clinical goals. The later studies had patients working on improvisations, psychodrama, musical games, and listening to and playing Cuban music. The findings for all studies showed a significant decrease in the use of medications among the patients who participated in the ongoing groups. These studies, while not perfectly controlled, marked the first research projects in Cuba addressing music therapy and mental health in geriatrics (Fernández de Juan, 2003).

MUSIC THERAPY AND HIPPOTHERAPY WITH CHILDREN WITH SPECIAL NEEDS

Music therapy with children was first addressed by Lic. Idida María Rigual González, who began to explore music therapy with children with special needs at the Regla Centro. González had also trained in hippotherapy, a form of therapy that uses the movements of horses, to help children with disabilities achieve better coordination. Working with children between the ages of eight months and nineteen years, she began a research project combining the two therapies. The children in her studies had diagnoses of Down syndrome, Rhett's syndrome, autism, cerebral palsy, and various motor disorders. By combining music-therapy techniques with hippotherapy, Rigual focused on psychomotor skills, sensory integration, and mental-health goals. Her findings are showing this integration of approaches to be a powerful combination, particularly with children with few verbal skills: both the music and the horses offer channels for nonverbal communication between the child and the therapist. The project has demonstrated results in areas of social and emotional development, sensory integration, and psychomotor skills, and is a part of a master's thesis being developed by Rigual (Fernández de Juan, Oliva Sánchez, & Rigual, 2007).

Domestic Violence Project

In Mexico, Fernández developed a music-therapy model for working with women affected by domestic violence. She brought this model to Cuba and has been working to raise awareness of the need for domestic-violence services. She is currently collaborating with the Federation of Cuban Women and other health providers to provide training in her model. This training would allow health workers to be "co-therapists" in their community health settings, bringing this work to the community level. In addition, Fernández and others traveled throughout the provinces in Cuba to lecture about music therapy to students and faculty at colleges and universities that offer degree programs in public health, as well as at health facilities that deal with domestic violence (Fernández de Juan, personal communication, November 29, 2007).

Hospital Psiquiátrico de La Habana

The Hospital Psiquiátrico de La Habana, is the country's psychiatric hospital most well known both in and outside of Cuba. It has been an innovative leader in the integration of both dance and music therapy in its occupational therapy programs for patients. The hospital's therapeutic dance program, known as *psicoballet*, is a therapeutic intervention based on ballet, dance, and therapy. Created in 1973 by the director of the Cuban National Ballet, Alicia Alonso, and psychologist Georgina Fariñas, it forms an important aspect of the occupational/arts therapy program at the hospital. *Psicoballet* programs are now in place in many institutions throughout Cuba and in some Latin American and European countries (Frank, 2005).

I was invited to observe a session of the program by dance therapist Ileana Freijes Tejera. The group I observed comprised primarily patients diagnosed with schizophrenia who were a broad range of ages and fitness levels. The sessions also incorporated music and percussion instruments. Many of the patients in the group attended this therapy daily. The hospital reports marked improvement for these patients in areas of social and emotional skills, and in the reduced dosages of psychopharmaceutical drugs necessary in their treatment. This reduction in the need for medication was striking. One of the common side effects of psychopharmaceutical drugs is a very noticeable impact on psychomotor ability and coordination. The *psicoballet* director and teachers described the gradual yet significant reduction in these side effects as patients participated in *psicoballet*. They reported that the negative psychomotor and coordination effects of these drugs were minimal to absent in the participating patients.

It was remarkable to observe the level of interpersonal interaction, physical interaction, peer support, and group cohesion (all areas of difficulty typical with this population) within the class. Group members carried themselves with strong posture that spoke of self-esteem and pride. During a rehearsal for an upcoming performance, those who were not yet ready to perform provided verbal feedback, constructive criticism, and support to other members. The class balanced the structure, discipline, and challenging technical demands of ballet with many opportunities for creative and emotional expression.

Music therapy that incorporates Cuban folkloric music is also an important component of the occupational therapy at the hospital. Participants include long- and short-term in-patients, day-treatment patients, and others, released from the hospital, who continue to return to participate in music therapy. The hospital has a long history of musical performance groups, including La Orquestra de los Pacientes del CUBA, which have played at national events, the Pan Am games, psychiatric conferences, and other events.

Music therapy at the hospital begins with the patients coming to the groups and listening. Interested individuals are slowly incorporated into the group and into active participation. The groups include both musicians and those with no musical experience. Some patients attend music lessons at music schools, and according to therapist Gloria Abad García: "Of course, they have just as much right to education as anyone else" (Abad García, personal communication, November 30, 2007). Musicians from the community also assist in the program.

A variety of music programs take place at the hospital, and they include very experienced musicians who are patients, as well as patients who are exploring music for the first time and learning to sing or play in bands. The patient groups use Cuban folkloric music and Cuban drumming, and they compete in *comparsas* (carnival bands and dance troupes) at gatherings at the hospital. All of these activities are part of a dedicated music-therapy program that performs regularly for visitors.

My Personal Vision of Intercultural Collaboration for the Future

Most striking about my experiences in Cuba has been the full circle of reciprocal learning and teaching that has taken place. I began visiting Cuba in 1994 to study percussion at a program at the Instituto Superior de Arte, a prominent music conservatory in Havana. I continued visiting to study with a variety of teachers and programs. At that time, no training programs in music therapy existed in Cuba, and it was a relatively unknown field. In 2000, as a music-therapy graduate student, I completed my research study on "The Therapeutic Aspects of Cuban Folkloric Drumming." The results contributed to my thesis, "Influences of Afro-Cuban Drumming on Percussion-Based Music Therapy." I applied that knowledge in my development of innovative percussion-based music-therapy approaches in the United States. I began to formulate and create percussion-based music-therapy methods that utilized musical applications of Cuban folkloric traditions, the therapeutic effects of drumming, and therapeutic aspects particular to group ensemble playing. I used these treatment approaches and methods in my work with children with special needs; children and adolescents with emotional and behavioral issues; and adults with HIV/AIDS, substance abuse, and psychiatric issues.

From the beginning of my research, I was surprised by my work's positive reception in Cuba. When I began the first study on the therapeutic aspects of Cuban folkloric music, I was unsure how it would be received, and wondered whether my questions and areas of interest would be relevant to the musicians. Everyone from traditional folkloric drummers to academic scholars expressed great interest and excitement about the topic, and several musicians felt it was an important area that they would be interested in pursuing and collaborating on further.

In 2001, after visiting the Centro de Salud Mental in Regla and observing their music therapy work with seniors and children, I began to meet informally to offer my assistance. I was invited by the director, Dr. Raúl Gil, to present at the Arts in Therapy Conference for the Central American and Caribbean region, a part of the larger Salumec Regla 2003 Mental Health Conference. This exposure led to my offering further presentations and teaching seminars at the Havana Bienel Arts in Therapy Conference, various mental health conferences, and the Instituto Superior de Arte.

I was continually impressed by the excitement and positive reception I received. It also intrigued me to discover which aspects of my work were most interesting and acceptable to the participants. Initially, there was great interest in my work with children, with a lesser response shown to my work with adults with HIV/AIDS and substance abuse. Interest began to increase as these issues became more openly discussed in Cuba. I also saw that—in a country where musical skill is so highly valued and competitive—a shift in perspective was required in order to use Cuban music as a therapeutic process without regard for the level of musical skill of the participants. What continually stood out, though, was the strong interest in my use of percussion and the way in which my methods were influenced by Cuban percussion. I was asked whether I would be willing to be interviewed, and was surprised when I learned that the interview was with Orfilio Pelaez for an article in the science and technology column of *Granma*, the newspaper of the Communist Party of Cuba. Individuals had been using Cuban music therapeutically, and at the same time the clinical field of music therapy was developing in Cuba; I began to see how my work represented the integration of the two. After seeing a presentation of my work at the Havana Bienel conference, Dr. Lorenzo Somarriba, the director of the Hospital Psiquiátrico de La Habana, invited me to visit and observe their *psicoballet* and music-therapy groups. This visit marked the beginning of another collaborative connection, with plans for further visits and sharing of our respective work. In 2008, I was invited to present my work at the new master's program at the University of Havana and Instituto Superior de Arte (ISA).

Throughout all my experiences in Cuba's community-health settings, it has been impressive to witness the talent, creativity, dedication, and resolve of the doctors, therapists, musicians, and mental-health professionals. Committed to developing their work regardless of personal gain or recognition, they persevere in spite of hardships, shortages, and difficult conditions. While Cuba looks to other countries to assist in developing its music-therapy profession, its own rich musical, cultural, and community-health traditions have a great deal to offer to the international music-therapy community.

Just as I found in my initial research study with musicians, the mental-health professionals and music therapists I encountered are eager for international exchange and collaboration. At the end of the *psicoballet* class with adults with schizophrenia, the patients shared their thoughts and experiences of the class with us. As one particularly articulate young man expressed, "I dream of the time when the embargo ends and we can come to your country and share with you this work that we are doing!" Everybody laughed with surprise, but beneath the laughter was a deep recognition that this work is important, that it needs to be shared, and how great such an exchange would be.

References

Chernoff, J. (1979). *African rhythms and African sensibility*. Chicago: The University of Chicago Press.

Crook, L. (1992). The form and formation of the Rumba in Cuba. In V. Boggs (Ed.), *Salsiology* (pp. 31–42). New York: Excelsior Music Publishing Company.

Fernández de Juan, T. (2003). Music therapy in Cuba: A brief journey to the immediate future. *Voices: A World Forum for Music Therapy*. Retrieved February 10, 2008, from http://www.voices.no/country/monthcuba_october2003.html

Fernández de Juan, T., Oliva Sánchez, R., & Rigual González, I. M. (2007). Update of music therapy in Cuba. *Voices: A World Forum for Music Therapy*. Retrieved January 21, 2008, from http://www.voices.no/country/monthcuba_october 2007.php

Frank, M. (2005). Havana to host International Congress of the Latin American Psychology Association. *MEDICC Review: Health and Medical News from Cuba*, December 2004. Retrieved February 17, 2008, from www.medicc.org/publications/medicc_review/1204/pages/headlines_in_cuban_health.html

González-Whippler, M. (1996). *Santería the religion*. St. Paul, MN: Llewellyn Publications.

Murphy, J. (1988). *Santería*. Boston: Beacon Press.

Nevis, M. (2001). *Influences of Afro-Cuban drumming traditions on percussion-based music therapy*. Unpublished master's thesis, New York University.

Peraza Chil, E., & Zaldívar Pérez, D. (2003). La musicoterapia: Un nuevo enfrentamiento al estés y la hypertensión arterial. *Revista Cubana de psicología*, 20(1), 10–22.

Puertas, G. (1975). La musicoterapia en ergoterapía y rehabilitación. *Revista Hospital Psiquiátrico La Habana*, 16(2), 229–242.

Shapira, D. (2002). New sounds in culture. *Voices: A World Forum for Music Therapy*. Retrieved February 17, 2008, from http://www.voices.no/columnist/col schapira110202.html

Sublette, N. (2004). *Cuba and its music*. Chicago: Chicago Review Press.

Uribe, E. (1996). *The essence of Afro-Cuban percussion and drum sets*. Miami, FL: Warner Bros. Publications.

PART V

Voices

CHAPTER EIGHTEEN

Assistance to Cuba's Jewish Community from International Jewish Organizations

David L. Strug

Jay Sweifach

Heidi Heft LaPorte

This chapter is about medical assistance and health-promotion programs funded and supported by international Jewish organizations and used by Cuba's Jewish community. In discussing this topic, it is important to consider demographic shifts in the Cuban Jewish community that resulted from the collapse of the former Soviet Union and also the effects of the U.S. trade embargo. These factors help us to understand the reason for support from the international Jewish community, especially from the United States. The loss of economic support stemming from the breakup of the former Soviet bloc had significant effects on the well-being of all Cubans, including those who are Jewish.

Health promotion and medical assistance by international Jewish organizations to members of Cuba's small Jewish community have helped to strengthen Jewish-community identity on the island. This aid has also promoted family cohesion and overall well-being in the Jewish community.

The aid given to the Jews of Cuba by international Jewish organizations reflects an important value embedded in traditional Jewish culture, that caring for the ill is the responsibility of all Jews. The assistance provided to Cuban Jews is likely to continue for the foreseeable future and at least for as long as the U.S.-imposed trade embargo on Cuba remains in existence. This embargo extends to medicines and most forms of medical assistance from the United States, and it also penalizes numerous other countries for offering such assistance to Cuba.

Cuba's Jewish population makes use of the same primary, secondary, and tertiary health-care services that are available to all Cubans as part of the government's national health system. However, the Jewish community also has access to medical assistance provided by Jewish international organizations. This assistance is targeted primarily, but not exclusively, at the Jewish population.

The information presented in this chapter is based on meetings held by the authors with twenty-nine members of the Jewish community on the island between 2003 and 2007. We held individual interviews and group discussions in both Havana and Santa Clara, the capital of the province of the same name located 160 miles east of Havana. Meetings were held in a variety of locations, including people's homes, public places, and in Jewish cultural and religious centers.

We asked respondents open-ended and semistructured questions about diverse aspects of Jewish religious and secular life, about their health-care needs, and about the type of health services they receive from the Cuban national health-care system and from international Jewish organizations. Our research methodology was qualitative. We tape-recorded and transcribed respondents' answers, coded the resulting transcriptions, and studied them to determine dominant themes.

Demographic Shifts in the Cuban Jewish Community

Ninety percent of Cuba's Jewish community left the island after the Cuban Revolution of 1959. The size of the Jewish community became so reduced after the revolution that it risked disappearing altogether.

The first Jews to come to Cuba in modern times arrived in 1898 as part of a U.S. expeditionary force during the Cuban War of Independence. About 1914, another wave of Jewish immigrants arrived from Turkey and Greece. In 1921, the United States passed the Emergency Quota Act, restricting immigration to its borders. European Jewish émigrés who were unable to gain entry into the United States began to settle in Cuba, many of whom would later attempt to emigrate to the United States. Thousands of Jews came to Cuba during the late 1930s, fleeing persecution from the Nazis. Most never became integrated into the Jewish community, and almost all of them left for the United States when the war ended.

In 1949, the Jewish population of Cuba numbered between ten thousand and twelve thousand persons (Levinson, 2006). By late 1965, only about 2,300 Jews remained (Levine, 1993). Those who did not leave were disproportionately older, poorer, and Turkish/Greek (Sephardic). The community, which had become vibrant, languished as a result of this exodus.

There is some uncertainty about the exact number of Jews living in Cuba today because many are not known to community leaders and are not counted in the official census. International Jewish agencies such as the Joint Distribution Committee (JCD) and Combined Jewish Philanthropies (CJP) estimate the number of Jews to be approximately 1,800. Today, there is a degree of out-migration of young Cuban Jews to Israel. This out-migration is offset to a certain extent by conversion of non-Jews through marriage to Jews.

It is important to note that the contemporary Jewish community has a disproportionately large number of older persons, as is the case for Cuba in general. However, this may be even more the case in the Jewish than in the non-Jewish community, since many young Jews have made aliyah, that is, have immigrated to Israel, while older Jews rarely leave the island. The Cuban government has, up to now, allowed Jews to leave Cuba for Israel, whereas emigration for most Cubans is severely restricted. The fact that there is such a high proportion of elderly Jewish Cubans has implications for health care, since older persons require more varied and more frequent health-care services than younger individuals.

International Jewish organizations have provided various kinds of support services for the Cuban Jewish community throughout the twentieth century. These institutions have included the Hebrew Immigrant AID Society (HIAS), the American Jewish Joint Distribution Committee (JDC or "el Joint"), the vocational/technical-training organization ORT (with a presence in Cuba since 1935), and the Jewish Joint Relief Committee (1937).

The Special Period

In the 1970s and 1980s, because of the U.S. blockade of the island, Cuba went through changes in its economy, including an increased economic dependency on the former Soviet Union. The collapse of the Soviet bloc in 1989 devastated the Cuban economy. It had a catastrophic impact on living standards and led to worsening economic and social conditions, including rising unemployment (Cole, 2002). Cubans call this time the "special period." During this time, most Cubans' income was insufficient to meet basic household needs (Togores González, 1999). Deteriorating housing and sanitary conditions resulting from limited availability of construction materials contributed to higher rates of disease. Dire economic conditions ensued for nearly a decade (Cooper, Kennelly, & Ordoñez-García, 2006). Food shortages during the worst phase of the so-called special period resulted in severely restricted monthly food rations, and many Cubans suffered from diseases caused by malnutrition and poor air quality. The health of the elderly was especially affected (Garfield, 1997).

The people we interviewed indicated that it was the period of time directly after the collapse of the former Soviet Union when there was an influx of humanitarian and medical assistance from Jewish organizations outside of Cuba because of the deteriorating socioeconomic conditions. One respondent spoke of his experiences during this time:

> The special period was a very, very bad period, very, very difficult. This was a difficult period for the whole population, but since we are talking about the Jews, let's concentrate on the Jews. For instance, Pesach [Passover] Jewish holiday stuff, which from the beginning had been donated by the Canadian Jews, well, they made a census of Jewish people in the '70s, and what happened was that it was such a difficult period that some families who had never been interested in Pesach products began to be interested because at least there was something that they could get. And then people began coming who hadn't previously identified as Jewish. I want this to be understood—it wasn't that this was an insincere thing, it just was that these people didn't come prior to that. It was really a difficult situation; in my case, I lost sixty pounds during the special period. People were really scared. They thought I had cancer. The doctor said no, it was just malnutrition.

The Trade Embargo

The U.S. trade embargo on Cuba has been in existence since 1962 and has limited the availability of medicines in the country. Cuba must pay higher prices for the medicines it imports because of transportation costs. This has caused a great deal of resentment in Cuba, especially when all Cubans are aware of the proximity of the United States, just ninety miles from the island. In 1991, Cuba's United Nations ambassador, Ricardo Alarcón stated that the "U.S. embargo has caused Cuba substantial material losses. Total prohibition of Cuba's acquisition of foodstuffs, medicine and medical supplies and equipment of United States origin . . . has caused and still causes appreciable additional harm to the Cuban people" (cited in Schwab, 1997, p. 16).

The combined effect of the U.S. trade embargo and the loss of subsidies from the Soviet Union created a shortage of medicine and medical equipment in Cuba. Although by design our interviews avoided political discussions, when talking about the lack of medication, one respondent indicated the embargo as a contributing factor in this shortage: "I hope someday you will end the embargo because the embargo only is doing badly—not for the government, but it is harmful for normal people to regular people. You see that they don't have medicine."

Health Care and Jewish Cultural Values

Commentators have noted that sanctity of life and life promotion are important themes in Jewish culture everywhere (Bonura, Fender, Roesler, & Pacquiao, 2001). Caring for the ill (*bikur cholim*), preservation of life (*p'kuach nefesh*), and taking care of the body (*shmirat haguf*) represent values that are embedded in the core teachings of Judaism. Jewish communities throughout the world have drawn on these values to guide behavior and action; so too have the Jews of Cuba. A high percentage of the people interviewed emphasized that the Jewish community has developed services and supports based on values such as those described above, with considerable aid coming from international Jewish aid organizations.

International Jewish Organizations and Medical Assistance

The Joint Distribution Committee has a long history of supporting vulnerable and at-risk Jewish communities throughout the world. The Cuban Jewish community owes much of its resurgence to the financial support and leadership provided by "el Joint." The JDC has provided spiritual leadership for the Jewish community of Cuba, funding for transportation to Sunday school and religious services, and funding for social and educational programs for children, adolescents, young adults, and seniors. With its support, many programs that address the health and well-being of the community have been developed, one example of which is an exercise program for seniors. The JDC has also been responsible for supporting community celebrations on the Jewish holidays and on the Sabbath.

The JDC has worked closely with the Jewish community through the offices of the Patronato de la Casa de la Comunidad Hebrea (Foundation of the Hebrew Community Home), or *el patronato* for short. The *patronato* was built in the Vedado district of Havana in 1949 to 1950 and was made up initially of primarily Ashkenazi Jews from Poland. Today the *patronato* represents the primary Jewish cultural, religious, and social institution in Cuba, and the office of the president of the Jewish community is located at the *patronato*. Dr. José Miller was the long-time president of the *patronato* and was a retired maxillofacial surgeon. He died in 2006, and William Miller, his son, currently serves as vice president. Representatives of international organizations that offer health promotion, and medical and other forms of assistance to the Jewish community typically work closely with *patronato* administrators.

The *patronato* also houses Cuba's largest synagogue, which is attended by both Sephardic and Ashkenazi Jews of all ages. For the Jewish community, the synagogue is the central venue for meeting both the spiritual and the practical needs of its members. One respondent noted the following about the Cuban synagogue: "We live in a society that lacks many necessities. The synagogue in one form or another, through donations outside, helps the individuals with medicine, with clothing, etc. It helps improve the person's educational, cultural, and technical sense of the capacity of themselves. The community has many intellectuals."

The assistance provided to the *patronato* and coming from international Jewish organizations is an important source of psychosocial support for the Cuban Jewish community. It helps maintain a variety of activities ranging from Hebrew classes for seniors to Israeli folk dancing for adolescents. These activities elevate the psychosocial well-being of hundreds of Jewish community members of all ages. The *patronato* also regularly sponsors outings for seniors to interesting places in Havana and elsewhere. We accompanied seniors on one such outing and were able to observe the happiness this trip brought group members.

The *patronato*'s cultural, religious, and social activities bring together family members of different generations and promote the cohesion of these families. This is an especially important function of the *patronato* given the fact that Cuban families typically live in multigenerational households and under crowded living conditions that can promote intrafamilial conflict (D'Angelo Hernández, 2008).

In 1991, with the assistance of the JDC, a free pharmacy was initiated at the *patronato*. According to one respondent, "The pharmacies in Cuba are poorly stocked, so this is a very important resource." The pharmacy, housed in a storage closet, has well-stocked shelves filled with prescriptions and over-the-counter medications, as well as vitamins, baby supplies, and other medical supplies. The pharmacy also stocks special medications completely unavailable in local pharmacies.

The pharmacy is managed by two volunteers: a retired gastroenterologist and her daughter, a pharmacist. It dispenses medication to Jews throughout the country and to non-Jews in the neighborhood. One person we interviewed noted: "We opened what you call a community pharmacy, because even though health care here is free, there is still a lack of a lot of medicines. We opened a community pharmacy upstairs, and we deliver medicine both to Jews and to non Jews." All persons requesting medications must demonstrate a verifiable medical need or have a prescription. The significant deficits in the availability of medication makes this service especially important.

Other organizations outside of Cuba, including the Canadian Jewish Congress, the Cuban Jewish Relief Project under the auspices of B'nai B'rith International, Hadassah International, and other visiting groups help stock the shelves, bringing medications to the pharmacy during trips to Cuba. The JDC has printed recommendations that are distributed to groups going to Cuba, asking travelers to bring medications and medical supplies.

The Cuban chapter of Hadassah International brings together Jewish health-care professionals in order to better meet the needs of the Jewish community. The chapter focuses on prevention of disease and presents community health-education programs on topics including first aid and prevention of diseases such as intestinal parasites, heart disease, stroke, and HIV/AIDS and other sexually transmitted diseases. There are lectures directed to both young children and seniors. For example, Rebecca Behar Tur, a volunteer working in the pharmacy, developed a program designed to provide health education and "starter kits" for mothers to help them care for their newborns and to supplement the assistance provided by the Cuban Ministry of Public Health. With the assistance of the international Jewish community, the program provides material assistance and guidance for the first six-to-twelve months of the child's life. Starter kits contain diapers, medicated creams and lotions, bottles, formula, over-the-counter baby medicines, clothing, and pamphlets about caring for newborns. These packages are delivered to each of the Jewish communities throughout the island. The chapter's health professionals maintain an ongoing relationship with the family and offer educational and emotional support in addition to material assistance.

Hadassah, an international women's Zionist organization, also provides health-education programs through games and contests to children of all ages who attend the Sunday school classes. The programs address issues ranging from healthy eating, dental hygiene, and the importance of washing hands for the younger children, to the prevention of sexually transmitted diseases and unwanted pregnancy for adolescents.

In addition, seminars about health care and nutrition are offered for Jewish seniors. Seniors are encouraged to participate in social activities organized by a JDC-funded program for members of the Jewish community over the age of fifty-five. These activities promote physical, mental, and social stimulation. The Hadassah chapter periodically offers special lectures and seminars for its members, many of whom are doctors and trained medical professionals. When possible, those with specialized medical training visiting from outside of Cuba are invited to provide lectures in their area of specialization.

The Cuban Jewish Relief Project of B'nai B'rith International (CJRP) was founded and is directed by its international chairman, Stanley

Cohen. It has provided assistance in identifying needs within the Jewish community and in providing financial support to meet those needs, many of which are health related. Medical technology is not as advanced in Cuba as it is in the United States and many other countries. There are unique cases in which a life-threatening disease cannot be treated because Cuba lacks the necessary medical equipment. One example we observed was the need for a suction machine to ease breathing for a five-year-old child suffering from Tay-Sachs disease. The Cuban Jewish Relief Project (CJRP) was instrumental in bringing this machine into Cuba as part of its humanitarian aid. Although the child was not Jewish, the Maimonides lodge (Cuban chapter of B'nai B'rith International), under the direction of its then president, the late Isaac Rousso, had the machine delivered to the child in Central Havana and arranged for a medical team to teach the family how to operate it. After the child's death, the machine was donated to a local hospital in Havana.

The Cuban Jewish Relief Project has been responsible for shipping hundreds of new wheelchairs to hospitals throughout Cuba, and for donating and delivering medical textbooks worth $500,000 to medical schools throughout the island. Beyond medical assistance and clothing, CJRP funds the Tzedakah Project. The Hebrew word *tzedakah* is based on a root meaning "justice" and in Judaism refers to the religious obligation to perform charitable and philanthropic acts, which Judaism considers important to living a spiritual life. The project provides a food allowance and supplemental income of $10 per month to disabled seniors to bring their income back up to pre-retirement levels. This amount of money represented approximately a third of the average monthly salary of a typical Cuban worker at the time of our research and is a significant supplement to the pensions given to Cuban seniors. In 2007, there were more than seventy individuals receiving this assistance each month. The Tzedakah Project also provides funding for the repair of severely damaged homes, which helps prevent health risk and injury due to unsafe living conditions.

The Future

One factor that may influence the degree to which international Jewish organizations continue to support medical assistance for Cuba's Jewish population in the future is the possible easing of travel restrictions between the United States and Cuba, now under discussion in the U.S. Congress (Cowan, 2008). The easing or elimination of these travel restrictions may result in much greater contact between the U.S. and Cuban Jewish communities. A diminution or elimination of travel restrictions is likely to result in an increase in the amount of medical assistance that international Jewish organizations provide Cuba's Jewish population. The Cuban government is also considering easing travel restrictions on trips abroad by its citizens (Boyle, 2008), which may promote medical assistance. As noted, Cuba generally permits its Jewish citizens to emigrate to Israel for religious reasons, but it is much more difficult to travel elsewhere in the world. An easing of travel restrictions would likely mean an increase in the number of Cuban Jews coming to the United States to seek help for serious medical problems. It might result in a greater permanent exodus of Cuba's Jewish population. The future is uncertain.

It is important to note that since the time of the revolution, the Cuban government has not interfered with the assistance provided by international Jewish organizations to meet the needs of Cuba's Jewish population. The Jews of Cuba have benefited from utilizing the nation's free and highly regarded health-care system, and they have been fortunate to also benefit from the health promotion and medical assistance programs made available to them through the *patronato*'s work with international Jewish organizations. We expect that assistance from these organizations will continue in its present form so long as the Jewish community of Cuba needs it and so long as travel restrictions on both sides of the Florida Straits remain.

References

Bonura, D., Fender, M., Roesler, M., & Pacquiao, D. F. (2001). Culturally congruent end-of-life care for Jewish patients and their families. *Journal of Transcultural Nursing, 12*(3), 211–220.

Boyle, C. (2008, April 18). Raúl Castro loosens travel restrictions for Cubans. *Daily News*. Retrieved June 18, 2008, from http://www.nydailynews.com/news/us_world/2008/04/18/2008-04-18_raul_castro_loosens_travel_restrictions_.html

Cole, K. (2002). Cuba: The process of socialist development. *Latin American Perspectives, 29*, 152–156.

Cooper, R. S., Kennelly, J. F., & Ordoñez-García, P. (2006). Health in Cuba. *International Journal of Epidemiology, 35*(4), 817–824.

Cowan, R. (2008, June 18). Congress panel votes to loosen Cuba travel rules. Reuters. Retrieved June 19, 2008, from http://www.reuters.com/article/politicsNews/idUSN1738649220080618

D'Angelo Hernández, O. (2008). Manejo de conflictos en la gestión comunitaria y las relaciones intergeneracionales. *Temas, 53*, 75–85.

Garfield, R. (1997). The impact of the economic crisis and the US Embargo on health in Cuba. *American Journal of Public Health, 87*(1), 15–20.

Levine, R. (1993). *Tropical diaspora: The Jewish experience in Cuba*. Gainesville, FL: The University of Florida Press.

Levinson, J. (2006). *Jewish community of Cuba: The golden years: 1906–1958.* Nashville, TN: Westview Publishing Company.

Schwab, P. (1997). Cuban health care and the U.S. embargo. *Monthly Review, 49*(6), 15–26.

Togores González (1999). Cuba: Efectos sociales de la crisis y el ajuste económico en los 90s. *Balance de la economía Cubana a finales de los 90s.* Habana: Universidad de la Habana CEEC.

CHAPTER NINETEEN

The Chinese-Cubans

Joyce Wong

"We are Chinese culturally, we are from China, understand?
But we live here in Cuba for a long time. It seems we now have
the Cuban culture, and then for the moment I have culture
from China and Cuba."
—Eighty-year-old Chinese-Cuban man

This work grew out of semistructured oral interviews conducted with nine elderly Chinese-Cuban men in Havana between January 2007 and April 2008. The author's strong interest in this community comes partly from her father's personal history as a Chinese immigrant to the United States and from her Latino (although not Cuban—her mother was born in Puerto Rico) background.

The Chinatown of today in Havana, known as *El Barrio Chino de la Habana en Calle Zanja,* is multigenerational, with thousands of Cubans claiming Chinese ancestry. Since the 1990s, when a shift in government policy allowed small private businesses to operate, many community groups have been working to revitalize the area. A Chinese-language newspaper, *Kwong Wah Po,* and a Chinese-language school, open since 1993, contribute to efforts to preserve Chinese culture in Cuba. Today, in addition to its role as a center for Chinese-Cuban culture, *El Barrio*

Chino is a tourist attraction where there are stores and restaurants that highlight the Chinese-Cuban experience.

It should be noted that the Cuban national health service, while open to all Cubans, does not consider people of a particular ethnic background as a special group (World Health Organization, 2005). Chinese-Cuban patients have equal access to health care, but like individuals of many other cultures, they also use traditional medicines and healing techniques in parallel with the mainstream Cuban health system. Traditional Chinese medicine is recognized, and homeopathy is taught in medical schools and in clinics, but their remedies are often not available in the state-run pharmacies. Further, the life-expectancy rate in Cuba is quite high, 77 years; and those over the age of sixty-five (10 percent of the population) are ethnically and racially diverse, and their numbers are increasing. The challenge for the Cuban health system is to identify and implement ways to keep this age group physically and mentally well.

A Brief History

Chinese-Cubans have become part of the social fabric not only of Cuba and the Caribbean but also of Latin America. Their stories are a testament to how they have managed to endure the traumas of bitter separation and solitude in a vastly different culture far from home. The personal experiences of Chinese-Cubans also demonstrate how entrepreneurial spirit and drive as well as close bonds with fellow Chinese immigrants on the island helped preserve their culture and identity even as age and immigration took heavy tolls on their community. Nearly a century ago, Cuba was home to one of the world's largest and most vibrant Chinese communities in the Western Hemisphere. Today, fewer than three hundred Chinese-born immigrants remain, many of whom are over age seventy.

The Chinese first arrived in Cuba in 1847 as contract laborers also known historically as "coolies," a racist term used to refer to Asians as slave labor. They were brought to fill the labor gap left by the gradual abolition of African slavery. From 1847 to 1874 about 125,000 Chinese laborers came to Cuba to work on the sugar plantations to satisfy the demand of the growing sugar industry.

During this period, 141,391 Chinese were transported by ship to Havana: 124,813 were sold and 16,576 died during the voyage. The mistreatment and atrocities committed against Chinese laborers were well documented with over a thousand depositions preserved in the *Cuban Commission Report* of 1896 (Helly, 1993). One excerpt illustrates extreme maltreatment: "We labor 21 hours out of 24 and [are] beaten . . . On one occasion I received 200 blows and though my body was a mass of wounds I was still forced to continue labor . . . a simple day becomes a year . . . and our families know not whether we are alive or dead." Wishing that in death they would return to their homeland, half of all suicides in Cuba in 1862 (173 out of 346) were committed by Chinese laborers (Thomas, 1971).

A second wave of Chinese immigrants also came to Cuba from the United States from 1860 to 1875, to escape the anti-Chinese and discriminatory legislation of California. These newcomers contributed to the economic stability that followed through the formation of businesses in the form of laundries, restaurants, and factories. Former laborers also joined the workforce as street peddlers.

A third wave of Chinese immigration came to Cuba from China after 1911 owing to the Chinese revolution. Chinese history in Cuba also includes the important role played by thousands of Chinese in the war for independence against Spain in the 1860s and 1870s, and as rebels and military generals who helped overthrow the Batista regime during the Cuban Revolution. After the triumph of the revolution in 1959, private businesses were nationalized, and there was a mass exodus of Chinese to the United States and Latin America. Those who remained, formed a small but vibrant community living in the larger cities in Cuba (Thomas, 1971).

The Interviews

The stories and themes that emerged from the interviews with these nine men offer insight and a glimpse into their daily lives and struggles. They show how these Chinese-Cuban men have been able to preserve their physical and mental health, maintain their sense of self, and find a place in the context of the Cuban health-care system and Cuban society. As many untold stories become lost or fragmented, this work became a genuine attempt to remember, capture, and document a small part of a link to individuals' connections to the Chinese diaspora. Personal narratives are and will always be a testament to a life lived and remain a powerful tool to understand the experiences of loss, displacement, and immigration and how they relate to the overall well-being and health of an individual. Recounting history allows for the preservation and conservation of historical memory of a group of people that have been underrepresented, marginalized, and perhaps misunderstood.

The nine oral interviews explore and capture descriptions of personal experience of overcoming and coping with adversity. Based upon recollections of and statements about the men's own feelings, the interviews revolved around questions about health practices and self-healing within the context of their Chinese identity. Interviews were based on a strengths-based paradigm that has been used to assess the process of self-healing (Mollica, 2006). Mollica (2006) proposes that the force of self-healing is a natural response to psychological illness and injury and is connected to the will to survive. The ability to heal past wounds and trauma for these Chinese-Cuban men was linked to their strong sense of ethnic and personal identity. The themes that emerged from the interviews included: (1) maintaining the Chinese identity and language, (2) health-related resources, and (3) self-healing and suppression of past traumatic experiences.

Maintaining the Chinese Identity and Language

The Chinese-Cuban men were all immigrants who arrived in Cuba as young boys and men. Several had families that had already established themselves on the island, while others had a more difficult time in making a place in Cuban society. All lived and kept their social networks within a Chinese community in and around Havana. One man, FL, age eighty-four, spoke of his family, which had arrived in Cuba in the late 1800s and had established a Chinese gambling casino. He did not come to Cuba until the 1930s and by that time his family were well-off and firmly established businesspeople. He describes his family's attempt to remain Chinese:

> My grandfather started a Chinese pharmacy. He brought Chinese foods into the country. He would say that many Chinese were missing their foods. It was for the Chinese that resided in Chinatown, so they would not miss their foods. There were Chinese natural medicines too! It was the first Chinese pharmacy, Chung Wong Tong, founded in 1910 on Calle Dragones, corner of Galiano. My father also had a broom factory, but it closed in 1942. Afterwards he opened a bodega, which remained open until businesses were nationalized after the revolution.

FL never married and lived among other Chinese-Cubans in Havana. He identifies as both Chinese and Cuban. He told the interviewer that before the revolution he was treated with disrespect. "They used to say I was stupid. You don't know anything! Everyone used to mess with the Chinese."

LB, a seventy-five-year-old Chinese-Cuban immigrant arrived in Cuba at age twenty. He too belonged to a family that had achieved economic success. In his words:

You cannot escape your Chinese identity in Cuba. I have Cuban citizenship, but naturally identify as a Chinese in Cuba. You always miss home very much. It was very hard without knowing the language, but luckily, my mother and my father were okay economically. I did not have to work and suffer. From the first year here I learned the language from the son of a Chinese. He would explain things for one year; I learned a little, then started working. Then it became easier to communicate with Cubans.

Other Chinese-Cuban men reported more difficult experiences adapting to Cuba and leaving China. Some of the men reported that as their families in Cuba became more established and secure, they experienced the adjustment process with less anxiety. Nevertheless, every person interviewed was keenly aware of their Chinese identity and had made efforts in their lives to maintain it. One man reported that he had no religious affiliations, and although he arrived in Cuba at age fifteen, he maintained a strong connection to the Chinese community, which remained an important resiliency factor for his whole life.

Health-Related Resources

As Cuban citizens, after the revolution, Chinese-Cubans (like everyone else) had access to free health care. Among the many obstacles they faced, language was a major challenge for them. Surely, they had been to the polyclinic to access health and dental services, but they volunteered little history about the details of their health-seeking behaviors. One man did complain that there was a lack of Chinese medicines in the Cuban pharmacies; but as a group, little else on the Cuban health system emerged. What was prominent was, as with many other immigrant groups, the experience of feelings of grief, loss, and assimilation to a new country. It was clear that some of the men might have met the criteria for clinical depression. For example, one man reported that he would endure feelings of sadness until he died, that death would relieve him of these feelings.

Self-Healing and Suppression of Past Traumatic Events

The concept of self-healing and the suppression of past traumatic events as a conscious coping mechanism were prevalent in the sample of Chinese-Cuban men. Traditional medicines, foods, spices, and teas were mentioned as central to their lives. The importance of the social network at the Chinese senior residence and Chinese senior center where these men met on a regular basis was underscored: "It is a better life here at the residence. I have Chinese comrades, we talk, converse here. I am well attended; I eat well and go walking outside." Another man stated: "I don't feel so alone because I always have company, and if I don't, I seek it, and then I am not alone. After lunch, three or four of us get together, because there are a few Chinese here, and then we go to play mah-jongg for the afternoon, without worries, not taking things to heart."

What did these men have to "take to heart"? First, with the exception of one man who lived with his wife and another who lived with his sister, they had all immigrated to Cuba leaving at least some family behind. Although one man mentioned a trip he had taken to Hong Kong, traveling for these men was not an option because of the expense and because of the visas that must be applied for in order to leave the country. It was clear that their most powerful resource was their connection with each other. The concept of self-healing applied, especially with regard to mood and emotional matters, and the strong bonds of kinship. The government-sponsored health system was utilized for serious health problems, but minimally. One eighty-five-year-old man's comment best sums up the philosophy held by these men regarding self-healing: "There are times when you just have to forget things for yourself; you have to look for happiness, and quit your thoughts."

Conclusion

The strong social support that these elderly men received and offered to others may counteract past adversity in their lives. The importance of social-support networks in ameliorating social isolation and improving overall physical and mental health and the quality of life is apparent for these men. According to Mollica (2006), self-healing is one of the human organism's natural responses to psychological illness and injury. The function of self-healing from the psychological dimension is its enhancement of the process of survival and recovery.

It is in this innate capacity to self-heal that these Chinese-Cuban men appear to have utilized strategies for coping by suppressing their feelings, memories of the past, and current stressors, which may explain their ability to adapt and recover from traumatic events in their lives such as leaving their homeland and the pervasive racism prior to the revolution. This resilience may be attributed to a protective factor of Chinese culture that is based on maintaining personal integrity, honor of the family, compassion, and interconnectedness to one another.

There have been many past stereotypes about the emotional world of Asians, which have been discredited in the last twenty-five years—for example, beliefs that Asians are not psychologically minded, that they do not benefit from group support, and present to health-care settings with somatic complaints. The interviews with the nine Chinese-Cuban men in Havana support the new scientific findings that Asians are indeed psychologically minded and receptive to mental-health interventions that are provided in a culturally competent manner. It can be concluded that the men remained emotionally and culturally resilient. Influenced by both Chinese and Cuban culture, they have constructed a worldview that allows them to respond to stress and past traumatic events with a strengths-based self-healing strategy. Their collective Chinese identity while living in Cuba seems to have helped them manage stress and live long lives. Self-awareness, control of emotions, and the enjoyment of each other's company seem to have had beneficial effects on their overall mental health and well-being.

References

Helly, D. (1993). *The Cuba commission report: A hidden history of the Chinese in Cuba* (first published in 1896). Baltimore: Johns Hopkins University Press.
Mollica, R. F. (2006). *Healing invisible wounds: Paths to hope and recovery in a violent world.* New York: Harcourt.
Thomas, H. (1971). *Cuba, the pursuit of freedom.* New York: Harper and Row.
World Health Organization. (2005). *Mental health atlas, 2005.* Retrieved on December 6, 2008, from http://www.who.int/mental_health/evidence/atlas/profiles_countries_c_d.pdf

---

My deepest gratitude to my colleagues James Lavelle, LCSW, and Dr. Richard Mollica from the Harvard Program in Refugee Trauma and to Ray Sanchez, Ousara Sophuok, Dr. Quinton Wilkes, Mirta Quesada, Dra. María Faguagua Iglesias, my parents, Fresdesbinda Tosado Wong and Wai Fai Wong, and all of my Cuban peers who helped me with this project.

CHAPTER TWENTY

Afro-Cuban Women and Health Care

María Ileana Faguagua Iglesias

Discrimination against Afro-Cubans has been long recognized by historians and to some degree continues today even when such behavior runs contrary to the principles of the Cuban Revolution. It is illegal to discriminate against any group in Cuba. However, the informal racial discrimination, to the extent that it may exist, can be expected to take its toll on Afro-Cubans, especially women facing gender and racial biases.

In order to combat discrimination, some Afro-Cuban women have taken to changing their appearance: wearing contact lenses to change their eye color, using hair extensions to change its texture, and using whitening creams on their skin. The belief for some is that being "white" has advantages in many venues.

The Cuban health system does not currently recognize race as a special category for treatment. This is so even when Cuban doctors have written on genetic variants that are likely responsible for different susceptibilities to disease. Equity, however, is not the same as equality, as in the case of Afro-Cuban women. Equal access to health care does not account for all the determinants of health that affect the physical and mental health of people. While it is true that there is equity in access to health services in Cuba that includes usage, quality, resource allocation, and financing, it is not the same thing as equality of health status, which is allocated more on the basis of one's race and/or gender.

Even if the Cuban system did offer differential health care to people depending on race, because of Cuba's history of encouraging mixed-race coupling, it would sometimes be difficult to determine what race a person belonged to, as appearance is not a scientific criterion. Nevertheless, there are illnesses that predominate among different groups, such as hypertension and diabetes among people of African descent. Cuban studies in the rural provinces in the east and west of the island have confirmed the high prevalence of these illnesses in places where the population is largely black.

Afro-Cuban women, like the rest of the island's population are legally entitled to benefit from access to the Cuban health-care system. This begins with visits to the "family doctor," usually just a few blocks from where they live, both in the large cities and in many rural communities. At the community doctor's office they are treated respectfully, like any Cuban in the neighborhood; and, as for all Cubans, there is typically a wait—sometimes a long one—for certain treatments.

Mental health is affected by the conditions of underemployment that many Cubans face. However, in Cuba, jobs where there is little or no discrimination are in the health-care sector. Doctors, nurses, and other health-care-provider jobs are open to women, and Afro-Cuban women are welcome in the ranks. Mental-health conditions are also affected by a person's living conditions. If an Afro-Cuban woman experiences domestic violence at home her mental state can be addressed, usually with a referral to the polyclinic. But many refuse to go, and those who do may get temporary help with their mood or anxiety, but the environmental problems remain the same. As in many countries, women who suffer from psychological and physical violence often keep it to themselves. In this way, the victims further victimize themselves, and although the Cuban health and mental-health system tries to accommodate them, it often does not succeed because it cannot change the social conditions in their lives.

If the Cuban health system did recognize racial differences there would still be a need to address other variables that affect health. I have already discussed discrimination, and adding to this problem are psychosocial factors including personality, education level, and socioeconomic status. It is also notable that in the typical Cuban family, the woman assumes most of the duties of child care and household chores, and they are less likely to get the type of exercise that is beneficial to the body. In Afro-Cuban families and other families as well, when you add on an ailing family economy, poor housing, inadequate food, and an increased possibility of problems with sons and daughters at risk for joblessness, pregnancy, and even prison, the stress is greater and can lead to illness.

The sexologist Mariela Castro Espín, director of the National Center for Sexual Health and Education, acknowledges the existence of prejudice and discriminatory attitudes, widespread in the population, in relation to anything that is identified as different and comments that the family is where attitudes and values are learned early on. Yet there remains insufficient research on how race, gender, and health are related within the context of prejudice and discrimination.

I have written of the social causes of disease and attribute many of the illnesses that Afro-Cuban women suffer from to their living conditions precipitated by racism and discrimination. I have stated that tensions from difficulties in family life for this group of women can bring about higher rates of hypertension and other illnesses. My thesis is that Afro-Cuban women may be subjected to higher levels of social pressure than other groups. Further, they often suffer in silence, fearing that talking about these issues will only create more discrimination and that they might be considered unpatriotic. This is of course unfair in that Afro-Cubans support the revolution, and many Afro-Cubans fought and later worked for its success. It is not my intention to be divisive, nor is it my view that the health system is flawed, but rather that the social cause of disease, especially for Afro-Cuban women, is an important area that needs more attention.

PART VI

Cuban International
Health Care

CHAPTER TWENTY-ONE

Cuba's Achievements in Promoting International Health

Grisell Pérez Hoz

*". . . only peace and cooperation among peoples will be able to
protect humanity from death . . ."*

—Fidel Castro Ruiz

In 1959, upon the triumph of the Cuban Revolution, there were 6,286
doctors in Cuba. Of this number, 50 percent emigrated, mostly to the
United States, including one-third of the professors from the only
medical school that existed in Cuba. In 1960, Chile suffered a great
earthquake that left thousands dead, and in spite of the recent massive
exodus of doctors and the political and economic instability that characterized the first years of the revolution, Cuba sent a medical brigade
and several tons of equipment and supplies to that country. This was the
germ of what in later years would grow into one of the most altruistic
programs of the Cuban Revolution: Cuba's program of medical cooperation with the rest of the world.

On May 23, 1963, the Cuban medical cooperation effort officially
began on an international level, when a brigade of health workers was
sent to Algeria. The group was composed of fifty-five members, and they
stayed fourteen months.

Since that time, Cuba has brought international medical cooperation
to more than fifty countries of Africa, the Americas, Eurasia, and the

Middle East. This cooperation effort has been characterized by human-ism, professionalism, and responsibility. Although Cuban cooperation in the field of health has been called a "political doctrine" by its detrac-tors, Cuba has maintained as an inviolable principle its willingness to offer assistance to all peoples and nations affected by natural disasters, grave epidemics, and other calamities, without reference to differences of ideology, creed, race, or culture. This aid has been offered while respecting the right of sovereignty of each nation, with Cuba espousing human solidarity as a duty and not an instrument of political influence. The altruistic deeds of Cuban men and women in "white coats" in Latin America, Africa, Asia, and Oceania have been innumerable.

Cuban medical cooperation has passed through different stages. In the decades of the seventies and eighties, its primary modality was the internationalist mission. A policy known as Compensated Cooperation was initiated toward the end of the eighties in those countries that lacked human capital in the field of health, but which had economic resources to compensate for this deficit. The direct-contract modality prevailed in the nineties, as in the case of the Republic of South Africa and Brazil, and toward the end of the decade, the Integral Health Pro-gram (PIS) [*Programa Integral de Salud*] came into being. In the new millennium, the development of the Bolivarian Revolution in Venezuela led to the development of the program *Barrio Adentro* (Mission into the Neighborhood), the most complete and advanced modality of health care offered in any country.

In response to Hurricane Katrina in August 2005, Cuba assembled 1,586 doctors to offer humanitarian assistance to the United States. The offer was declined. On September 19, 2005, Fidel Castro created the Henry Reeves International Contingent of Doctors Specializing in Dis-asters and Serious Epidemics. This contingent lends support in cases of natural disasters and in epidemics with disastrous health and social consequences, such as in the case of HIV/AIDS and dengue.

Among the principal functions performed by Cuban international cooperation are the following: clinical/surgical medical assistance in the most remote and difficult geographical regions of a country, the development of health-education campaigns and mass vaccinations of the population, hygienic/epidemiologic inspections, and the donation of services to victims of disasters and other unforeseen emergencies. The greatest expression of Cuban international cooperation was demonstrated after Hurricanes George and Mitch passed through vari-ous countries of Central America and the Caribbean in 1998, leaving in their wake more than thirty thousand dead and untold damage to the health-system infrastructure of these countries.

In view of the gravity of the situation, Cuba immediately responded with the deployment of medical and paramedical personnel for as long as they were needed, with medicines and technical equipment. Cuban medical brigades reacted with the urgency that the situation called for: the first brigades went to Honduras on November 3, 1998; to Guatemala on November 5, 1998; to Nicaragua on November 12, 1998; and to Haiti on December 4, 1998. Subsequently, some of these countries requested that their Cuban collaborators remain.

The Integral Health Program emerged as a modality to bring free medical services to countries in need. PIS is characterized not only by the offer of medical services, but also by its development of human capital in the health-services sector. The strongest example of this cooperation is found in the Latin American School of Medicine (ELAM) created February 27, 1999, which was an expression of the political will of the Cuban government to continue contributing to the development of health professionals in countries that lacked an adequate number of health-care workers. This is necessary because the World Health Organization (WHO) has estimated that four million health-care personnel are lacking throughout the world. Special help is being given to Third World countries, which have an infant-mortality rate on average twenty times greater than in the developed countries, thirty years less life expectancy, and one hundred times fewer qualified health-care personnel. These differences can only be resolved through effective action and by means of international cooperation.

The fundamental mission of ELAM is to produce doctors with scientific and technical expertise, who practice medicine in a highly ethical manner, and in whom there prevails a spirit of humanism, human solidarity, and internationalism. ELAM is another contribution of Cuba in achieving sustainability in the health-care systems of other countries.

The priorities of the Integral Health Program are the integration of health care at the primary and secondary levels, technical assistance, the formation and support of human capital in health care, the development of health programs, and the management of medication programs.

The Integral Health Program provides to countries in need (at no cost) a health collaborator, especially a family doctor (*médico general integral*), for a period of two years, who offers services in rural areas and in areas of difficult access without interfering in the work of the doctors of the country. The host country provides transportation for the personnel involved and provides a stipend, food, and lodging. The health collaborators are not involved in internal political affairs, and they respect the laws and customs of the places where they lend their services. Medical attention is provided to the entire population without distinction of race, creed, or ideology.

Cuban health collaborators, doctors, nurses, and health technicians, work in the most remote areas of Latin America, the Caribbean, Central and South America, as well as in countries in Africa and Asia. Their work demonstrates how much can be done despite economic limitations and the impact of the blockade imposed by the United States. As Fidel Castro has noted, ". . . the Integral Health Program cannot be measured only by the number of lives saved, but by the millions of people who basically feel safe."

By the end of 2005, the Integral Health Program had saved more than a million lives and carried out more than sixty-six million medical consultations, thirteen million in homes located in poor communities that are difficult to access. Vaccination campaigns supported by the WHO provided almost nine million doses of vaccine. This contributed to diminishing infant and maternal mortality. In Gambia, the infant-mortality rate of 121 per 1,000 individuals was reduced to 40.6 per 1,000 with the help of the Cuban collaborators.

The pillar of the Integral Health Program is primary medical care (APS), which has an integrated biopsychosocial, preventive as well as curative, rehabilitative, clinical, epidemiological, and social focus. This new program of medical training occurs at the service sites of the national health system, with special emphasis on the APS work sites; hands-on education in the workplace is the fundamental training process. A graduate of the School of Medicine is a general primary doctor (MGB) able to do the following:

- Provide medical attention to children, adolescents, adults, pregnant women, and the elderly individually, in the family context, and in social circles through promotion, prevention, attention, and rehabilitation, and in their physical, psychological, and social aspects.

- Detect negative environmental effects and carry out programs of hygiene in the community and in the school setting to protect the health of the individual, the family, and the community.

- Carry out administrative functions to permit an efficient utilization of human, material, and economic resources under his or her responsibility, as well as assess and evaluate health programs.

- Provide health education to individuals, families, and the general population.

- Participate in his or her own education and in that of health workers on a technical as well as pre- and postgraduate level.

- Master the basic tools of scientific research to develop studies in the work environment.

- Carry out medical attention of individuals in case of disasters of any sort, and prepare the population in medical/sanitary aspects.

The general primary doctor on completion of his or her postgraduate work as a specialist in integral general medicine (more commonly called family medicine) is capable of providing international medical cooperation in any location as a result of his or her scientific and humanistic training.

The majority of collaborators in Cuba's medical brigades are specialists in integral general medicine, but, many of these doctors also hold a second specialty such as internal medicine, obstetrics and gynecology, pediatrics, anesthesiology, or cardiology.

Cuban doctors receive specialized training before leaving for the country where they will lend their cooperation. This training includes courses in foreign language (English or French) according to the official language of the country where they will lend their services; tropical diseases; disaster and grave-epidemic medicine; natural and traditional medicine; geography; the habits, customs, and idiosyncrasies of the affected population; economic and social systems; and statistical and demographic facts related fundamentally to the analysis of the health situation and health indicators of the country in question. At the start of Cuba's medical cooperation program, Cuban help was essentially medical assistance, but over time has become combined with the development of technicians and consultants for different ministries of health and of community leaders. For example, it is not unusual to see a Cuban physician in different parts of Africa or Central America training the religious leader of the community in the use of medicinal plants.

With the startup of new medical-training programs, international educational work has assumed an ever-greater importance in those countries where Cuba sends medical assistance. The opening of medical schools abroad with Cuban personnel in such places as South Yemen in 1975, Guyana in 1984, Guinea-Bissau in 1986, Gambia in 2000, Equatorial Guinea in 2000, and Eritrea in 2003, to cite only a few examples, constitutes a commitment on Cuba's part to guarantee true sustainability. Sustainability is understood in the context of Cuban medical cooperation as the possibility that the country that receives Cuban aid will have capable medical personnel and dozens of new national doctors who will occupy the posts once held by their Cuban collaborators when those collaborators leave.

A new type of cooperation arose in 2003 with the deployment of a medical brigade to Venezuela, composed of professionals who had participated in earlier missions through the PIS. The program *Barrio Adentro* [Mission into the Neighborhood] was initiated, whereby the doctor is in the center of the community in the poorest and most abandoned locations. The development of human capital as part of the work of the Cuban medical brigades in the *Barrio Adentro* program has been very meaningful and is founded on the following principles:

- Health as a social right

- Primary health care

- Quality of life

- Promotion of health and disease prevention

- Citizen participation

The objectives of this program are to help achieve appropriate social relevance for the future doctor within his or her community; to promote the integration of the teaching, service, and research aspects of the doctor; and to inculcate in medical students a heightened social and humanistic sensibility and commitment to the society from which they come and where they will work once trained.

On the international stage, the program attempts to prepare physicians in a holistic manner. Physicians must be prepared from the cognitive/affective point of view with the qualities and sentiments that will be needed in the course of their career to promote health, prevent disease, and to rehabilitate the patient physically and socially. Physicians must be prepared to work with a perspective that is above all else humane, in a manner that is ethical, scientific, and technically proficient so that they may keep up with the times and possess knowledge of advances in the field of health. The physician must be prepared so that he or she may be a well-trained doctor, with the spirit of commitment to the most noble and human of callings, that of saving lives and keeping watch over the health of the community. The overall goal is for the professional to be competent, honorable, internationalist in orientation, ethical, forthright, responsible, honest, and for the physician to practice with the conviction that ". . . a better world is possible."

Reference

Castro Ruiz, F. (2002). Discurso pronunciado en el acto conmemorativo por el aniversario 40 del Instituto Superior de Ciencias Básicas y Preclínicas Victoria de Girón, October 17, 2002.

Index